Is It Alzheimer's?

A Johns Hopkins Press Health Book

Is It Alzheimer's?

---

101 ANSWERS TO YOUR MOST PRESSING QUESTIONS ABOUT MEMORY LOSS AND DEMENTIA

Peter V. Rabins, MD, MPH

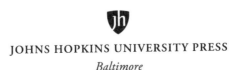

JOHNS HOPKINS UNIVERSITY PRESS

Baltimore

Note to the Reader: This book is not meant to substitute for medical care and treatment should not be based solely on its contents. Instead, treatment must be developed in a dialogue between the individual and his or her physician. Our book has been written to help with that dialogue.

Drug dosage: The author and publisher have made reasonable efforts to determine that the selection of drugs discussed in this text conform to the practices of the general medical community. The medications described do not necessarily have specific approval by the US Food and Drug Administration for use in the diseases for which they are recommended. In view of ongoing research, changes in governmental regulation, and the constant flow of information relating to drug therapy and drug reactions, the reader is urged to check the package insert of each drug for any change in indications and dosage and for warnings and precautions. This is particularly important when the recommended agent is a new and/or infrequently used drug.

© 2020 Johns Hopkins University Press
All rights reserved. Published 2020
Printed in the United States of America on acid-free paper
9 8 7 6 5 4 3 2 1

Johns Hopkins University Press
2715 North Charles Street
Baltimore, Maryland 21218-4363
www.press.jhu.edu

Library of Congress Cataloging-in-Publication Data

Names: Rabins, Peter V., author.
Title: Is it Alzheimer's? 101 Answers to Your Most Pressing Questions about
    Memory Loss and Dementia / Peter V. Rabins, MD, MPH.
Description: Baltimore : Johns Hopkins University Press, 2020. | Series:
    A Johns Hopkins Press Health Book | Includes index.
Identifiers: LCCN 2019015979 | ISBN 9781421436395 (hardcover : alk. paper) |
    ISBN 1421436396 (hardcover : alk. paper) | ISBN 9781421436401 (pbk. : alk.
    paper) | ISBN 142143640X (pbk. : alk. paper) | ISBN 9781421436418
    (electronic) | ISBN 1421436418 (electronic)
Subjects: LCSH: Alzheimer's disease—Miscellanea. | Dementia—Miscellanea.
Classification: LCC RC523.2 .R33 2020 | DDC 616.8/311—dc23
LC record available at https://lccn.loc.gov/2019015979

A catalog record for this book is available from the British Library.

Special discounts are available for bulk purchases of this book. For more information, please contact Special Sales at 410-516-6936 or specialsales@press.jhu.edu.

Johns Hopkins University Press uses environmentally friendly book materials, including recycled text paper that is composed of at least 30 percent post-consumer waste, whenever possible.

Note to the Reader

Is It Alzheimer's? is not intended for use as medical or legal advice and should not be used in that way. Individuals should always ask their medical practitioner and lawyer about questions they have about their own care or, when authorized, about the care of other people.

This book contains discussions of the off-label use of medications. This means that some medications are discussed that have not been approved for that use by the Food and Drug Administration. These discussions are not intended to be an endorsement of the use of these medications. Rather, these discussions describe how medications are prescribed by some practitioners and describe whether there is scientific evidence supporting their use.

Peter Rabins has received no financial support from pharmaceutical companies in the past 5 years.

Contents

Preface

This book answers 101 of the most common questions I am asked about Alzheimer disease and other dementias. It was written to supplement *The 36-Hour Day*, which Nancy Mace and I first published almost 40 years ago.

Readers who find this book helpful but want more information should turn to *The 36-Hour Day*. It has more detail on the 4 central themes of this book: information on the diseases that cause dementia; tips on how to improve the quality of life of people with dementia and manage the symptoms caused by the disease; suggestions for caregivers about steps they can take to improve their psychological and physical well-being; and a summary of some recent research advances.

The 36-Hour Day and *Is It Alzheimer's?* both use the labels "Alzheimer disease," "Parkinson disease," and "Huntington disease" without an apostrophe after the name of the person credited with first describing the disease. I (and some others) omit the apostrophe because it implies that the disease belongs to the doctor who first described it. I have also chosen to use the term "caregiver," even though alternative words and phrases have been suggested. Each of the alternatives also has limitations and "caregiver" is still the most widely used term in the United States.

Some of the questions I answer address issues about which experts disagree. I have tried to indicate when this is the case so that the reader will know that I am expressing an opinion that knowledgeable experts may disagree with. Such disagreements are inherent to the discussion of any issue about which there is ongoing research and a consensus has not emerged.

Two examples of such issues are the prevention of dementia and the cause of Alzheimer disease.

For 40 years I have had the extraordinary gift of knowledgeable and supportive teachers and colleagues. Many of the answers in this book are informed by what they have taught me. Likewise, many answers in the book can be traced to information I have learned from patients and caregivers. I am indebted to all those who have contributed in this way, but I take full responsibility for any errors. I have also been the beneficiary of financial support from the T. Rowe and Eleanor Price Foundation, the Richman Family Professorship for Alzheimer Disease and Related Disorders at Johns Hopkins University, the Stempler Fund for Dementia Research, the National Institute of Mental Health, the National Institute on Aging, the National Institute of Neurological Disorders and Stroke, and many individual donors. This support has been crucial to my efforts in public education, including this book.

Is It Alzheimer's?

Should I Worry about My Memory?

___

Q1. What happens to memory and thinking as we age?

___

A1. Beginning in our 30s or 40s, the retrieval of information that we know, especially names and words, becomes more difficult. This ability is sometimes referred to as "free recall memory," because it is our attempt to report, in words and without clues, knowledge we have stored in our brain. Research has shown that the average 25-year-old can recall between 6 and 7 words from a list of 10 unrelated words read to them several minutes before. The average 75-year-old, in contrast, recalls about 5 words from that list. This means that *free recall memory declines* as we age, even though the change is not dramatic.

The results are different if you change the experiment. The study starts out the same, giving people a list of 10 words to remember. But rather than ask them to recall as many words as they can after the several-minute delay, the researcher gives them a written list of 20 words, 10 of which are the words they were asked to remember and 10 of which are new words. When asked to circle only the 10 words they were initially asked to remember, the 75-year-olds and the 25-year-olds do equally well. This indicates that the ability to correctly recognize previously encountered information, *recognition memory*, is *not affected* by normal aging. The different results from these two studies demonstrate that normal aging is not accompanied by a decline in *every* type of memory.

In addition, *speed of performance*, both physical and mental, slows as we age. This means that putting pressure on older people to perform quickly puts them at a disadvantage. If given enough time, older people perform normally on many tests.

Q2. I am having trouble remembering the names of friends and family members and difficulty coming up with the words I want to say. Should I worry?

A2. The definition of dementia requires *both* a decline in thinking (also called "cognition") and a decline in the ability to perform everyday activities such as work routines, household activities, and using transportation. If you have not had a decline in daily functioning as a result of cognitive change, then you do not meet criteria for dementia.

Recognition memory, the ability to correctly remember previously encountered information when given a yes-no choice, does not appear to be affected by normal aging.

However, when the symptoms of dementia are first developing, there is a period in which daily functioning is not yet affected. This condition is called "mild cognitive impairment (MCI)." It is defined as a decline in memory or one other cognitive ability (for example, judgement or following directions) of 30% to 45%. At present, testing by a neuropsychologist is the best way to determine if there has been this degree of decline.

Neuropsychologists administer tests that determine what a person's lifelong abilities have been and tests that measure whether there has been a decline from that level. People who have persistent worries about their memory, who are told by others who know them well that they are repeatedly forgetful or not performing at their usual level, or who believe that their thinking problems are interfering with their daily lives should be tested by an expert. Neuropsychological testing is time consuming and expensive, and is administered by experts who are not available in every community. This is one reason why scientists are trying to identify blood tests or other biological measures (referred to as "biomarkers") that would identify those who should undergo in-depth testing.

An expert in the assessment of cognition should test a person who
- has persistent worries about their memory;
- has been told by others who know them well that they are repeatedly forgetful or not performing at their usual level; or
- believes that their thinking problems are interfering with their daily lives.

Q3. Are there benefits to the early recognition of mild cognitive impairment (MCI) and dementia?

A3. Most experts believe that early identification of MCI and dementia will encourage people to write a will and designate a durable power of attorney for health (*see Q59*) if they have not already done so. Early identification might help people begin to make necessary changes in their lives. It might also help loved ones or others close to the person realize that changes they are observing are due to a disease that is impairing thinking, not to purposeful resistance or psychological difficulties. None of these potential benefits has been proven. I have been told by some people that they would want to know as soon as possible if they are developing dementia, but others have said that they would not want to know their diagnosis early unless there were a definitive treatment. In my opinion, universal screening should become the norm only if it improves patient outcomes or if disease-modifying treatments are available.

———

Q4. I live alone and am concerned about my memory. For a few years I have had intermittent trouble remembering things, but so do my friends. I mentioned this to my primary care doctor on my last visit and she reassured me that there was nothing to worry about. Now I'm worried because I've started having trouble doing my checkbook, something I have always done without difficulty, and last year I needed to get help filling out my tax forms, another thing I had always done myself. Should I be evaluated? If so, should I go to a memory specialist?

———

A4. Word-finding difficulty or occasionally misplacing keys or glasses does become more common as people age (*see Q1*), but difficulty doing activities that were previously within a person's capabilities, such as filling out a checkbook, banking online, filing taxes, cooking meals, and being effective at work, does not. I'd suggest you contact your primary care doctor and tell her about your new symptoms. In general, primary care physicians are capable of evaluating people for dementia, but when a person is young (under age 65), has developed difficulty thinking over a period of weeks or months, or has developed signs of neurological disease such as weakness, tremor (shaking), muscle twitching, or numbness in the hands or feet, the person should see a specialist in dementia. I suggest discussing with your primary care doctor whether she can evaluate you or would prefer to refer you to a knowledgeable specialist.

2

What Is Dementia?
What Is Alzheimer Disease?

Q5. What is dementia?

A5. "Dementia" is an umbrella term that refers to any disease that has these 4 characteristics:

1. Begins in adulthood

2. Causes decline in 2 or more aspects of thinking (such as memory, organization of information, language, math, perception, judgement)

3. Causes a decline in the ability to carry out at least one activity of everyday life related to self-care, work, or independence

4. Does not impair level of alertness or ability to pay attention

There are 100 or more diseases that cause dementia. All meet these 4 criteria, but they differ in the specific aspects of thinking they impair, in the neurological symptoms they cause, in how rapidly they progress, in what causes them, and in how they are treated.

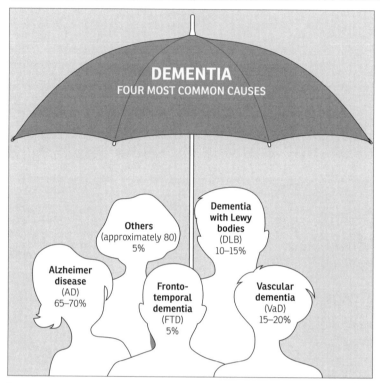

There are more than 99 causes of dementia. The 4 most common are Alzheimer disease, Lewy body dementia, vascular dementia, and frontotemporal dementia.

Alzheimer disease is the most common cause of dementia. The diagnosis of *definite* Alzheimer disease requires evidence of the specific changes in the brain described in *Q7*, but when a doctor uses the following criteria when assessing a patient, the diagnosis agrees with what is found later, at autopsy, more than 90% of the time:

1. A **slowly progressive dementia**, which means that the person has had slowly worsening memory or other cognitive (thinking) difficulties for more than 6 months.

2. **Lack of evidence of any of the other 99 causes of dementia** after physical, neurological, and psychiatric examinations, and on laboratory testing and brain imaging.

3. The presence of **memory impairment** *plus* **at least one of the following**:

   • impairment in executive function (abstraction, judgement, initiation, and persistence and stopping of thought or action);

   • impairment in language expression (called "aphasia");

   • impairment in doing everyday activities (called "apraxia") that is not attributable to impaired strength or sensation;

   • impairment in accurately perceiving the world visually (called "visual agnosia").

4. If under age 70, **a positive amyloid PET scan or spinal fluid markers** supporting the presence of Alzheimer disease.

Q6. Does every case of Alzheimer disease begin with memory impairment?

A6. While the vast majority of people with Alzheimer disease have difficulty remembering new information as their first symptom, not everyone does. Occasionally, the first symptom is difficulty finding and expressing words (*see Q18*), difficulty accurately perceiving the world around them, declining ability to function at work or home (*see Q8*), or apathy.

Q7. Is it true that Alzheimer disease can be diagnosed only at autopsy?

A7. If the doctor follows the criteria described in *Q5*, then autopsy confirms the diagnosis of Alzheimer disease made during life about 90% of the time. In the remaining 10%, one or several of the other diseases that cause dementia are present. It is likely that some combination of amyloid PET scan (*see Q9*

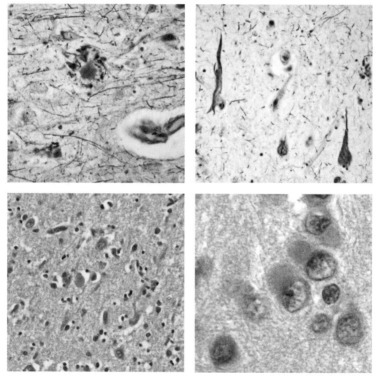

Microscopic findings in 3 diseases that cause dementia. Neuritic plaque (*top left*) and neurofibrillary tangles (*top right*) are characteristic of Alzheimer disease, cortical Lewy bodies (*bottom left*) are characteristic of dementia with Lewy bodies, and Pick bodies (*bottom right*) are characteristic of frontotemporal dementia (FTD). Courtesy of Dr. Richard E. Power and Dr. Olga Pletnikova.

and Q10), tau PET scan, or spinal fluid measures of amyloid and tau breakdown products will improve the accuracy of diagnosis made during life in the near future, but the usefulness of such testing has not yet been proven.

At autopsy, Alzheimer disease is characterized by abnormal structures called "neuritic plaques" and "neurofibrillary tangles" that are found in specific areas of the brain. The plaques consist of a core of *amyloid protein* surrounded by a mixture of the breakdown products of brain cells. They are located in the tissue *between* cells. The tangles consist of twisted fibrils of the protein *tau*. These are located *within* cells. *Q26* discusses these structures in more detail.

Q8. I have heard that there are stages of Alzheimer disease. How are they identified?

A8. There are several widely used descriptions of how Alzheimer disease progresses. Each has strengths and weaknesses. I favor a 3-stage model that was first described in the early 1950s.

Significant variability occurs in all diseases, so any description of staging must be understood as a broad generalization. The average person with Alzheimer disease lives about 10 years, and each stage averages about 3 years in duration. However, some people go from first symptom to death in 3 or 4 years and others live for more than 20 years.

Stage 1: Memory and Executive Function Impairment

People in this stage have difficulty learning new information but remember information from the more distant past. People also have difficulty organizing more complicated activities and may make subtle social errors. *Executive function* refers to a set of abilities that are crucial to organizing life. They include knowing when to start, continue, change, and stop an activity, as well as the abilities to abstract, generalize, and detect social cues.

People in this stage often remain independent, but their ability to do so declines as the disease progresses. People should be encouraged to continue doing activities they have always enjoyed, to participate in family events, and to remain socially active as long as there is no significant risk of harm to them or others. Some people are able to work but may require increased supervision.

Stage 2: Cortical Symptoms

This stage is characterized by impairments in 3 distinct aspects of cognition: language, praxis, and visual perception. Since people vary in the extent to which each capacity is impaired, it is important to identify each individual's remaining abilities and limitations in each. The symptoms of this stage are referred to as "cortical" because these functions of the brain are located in the outer layer of the brain, the cortex.

Language: People with Alzheimer disease can develop problems both expressing themselves with words and understanding what is being said to them. These language impairments are referred to medically as "aphasia." They are similar to what happens when people have a stroke or other injury in the brain's language area.

These impairments in language make it difficult for people to express what they want to say. People with aphasia will sometimes say a word they do not mean to say, will sometimes

Communication with a person who is having trouble expressing and understanding spoken language can often be improved by:

- speaking in short phrases or sentences rather than in long, complex sentences,
- succinctly repeating what you have said or asked,
- using nonverbal communication, such as visual cuing (pointing, for example) and touch, and
- asking them to do one task at a time rather than making requests involving multiple steps.

say words that have no meaning, or will not be able to express what they want to say. Aphasia can result in a person's being unable to answer questions accurately. For example, the person might not be able to say that they are in pain or to describe when and where it hurts.

People who are unable to understand what is said to them will have difficulty following directions. This can be tested for by asking them to carry out a multistep request. For example, if asked to "Please take the dishes into the kitchen and bring out the dessert," they may do one step but not the other or may just stare at the person making the request.

Communication with a person who is experiencing an aphasia, or language impairment, can often be improved by speaking in short phrases or sentences rather than in long, complex sentences; succinctly repeating what you have said or asked; using nonverbal communication, such as visual cuing (pointing, for example) and touch; and asking the person to do one task at a time rather than making requests that involve multiple steps. Speech-language pathologists, psychologists, nurses, and doctors can help identify ways to improve communication with a specific individual.

Praxis: The word "apraxia" refers to the inability to carry out a learned physical (or "motor") activity even though strength and sensation are normal. Examples include difficulty dressing, cooking, bathing, and using eating utensils. Like all symptoms in Alzheimer disease, these impairments develop gradually. A person may still be able to do parts of the activity but not the most complicated aspects of it. For example, a person may be able to put on pants or a blouse but not be able to put on a belt or bra, or use a zipper.

When observing a person with an apraxia, you can often figure out what they can still do on their own and what they need help with. If a person is having difficulty dressing, for example, observe whether they can put on slacks but not a belt.

The goals of helping people with impaired abilities are to maximize their independence while simultaneously helping them accomplish what they cannot do on their own. For example, a person developing difficulty using eating utensils will gradually lose these skills over months or years. The most complex task is using a knife, while the simplest is using a spoon. For people developing difficulty using a knife but still able to use other utensils, cutting their food in the kitchen before bringing it to the table will enable them to feed themselves with a fork and spoon. This means they are fully independent. Since there is no knife at their place setting, you have also helped them avoid the utensil they have difficulty with.

"Talking people through" tasks they are having difficulty with—that is, explaining each step as you go—may calm them and allow them to accept help with dressing, bathing, getting up from a chair, and feeding themselves.

Visual Perception: People with Alzheimer disease gradually develop difficulties in several aspects of visual perception. These impairments are called "agnosias." Some people with agnosia are unable to recognize familiar faces or places. Others are unable to observe more than one thing at a time even though there are several objects in front of them. For example, they may report that there are only peas on a plate when there are also several other items on the dish. People with agnosias might recognize people by their voices but not by looking at them.

> The goal of helping people with impaired abilities is to allow them to do everything they can while helping them accomplish what they cannot.

Being unable to recognize familiar places means that the person can never be in a familiar environment. This is a common source of distress in people with dementia, but hugging the person, engaging them in conversation, and finding activities they are able to enjoy can help them feel connected.

Stage 3: Physical Decline

Problems in walking, controlling urination and bowel movements, and swallowing develop gradually in this stage. People do not necessarily develop all of these impairments, and it is not possible to determine who will and will not develop any of them.

People with stage 3 symptoms need more physical support. They may need help with toileting and walking. As the stage progresses, food may need to be cut in very small pieces or pureed to aid in swallowing. Falls become common and some people lose the ability to walk.

Q9. How do brain scans work? Can they detect dementia and specific causes of dementia?

A9. Brain scans rely on a variety of atomic particles to visualize the contents of the brain. Standard X-rays can distinguish bone from water, but they do not visualize brain tissue, because it is mostly water.

CT scans of the brain take multiple X-ray pictures from different angles. A computer program then takes this information and generates a picture of the soft tissue of the brain and of the bones of the skull.

MRI scans use a strong magnet to generate a very brief magnetic field. This "lines up" water molecules and results in an image that can be captured on a computer screen. MRI scans can directly visualize brain tissue, flowing blood, and actively working brain cells.

Neither CT scans nor MRI scans can diagnose Alzheimer disease. They can detect old and new strokes, brain tumors, brain abscesses, normal pressure hydrocephalus (NPH), and subdural hematomas (collections of blood between the lining of the brain and brain tissue which press on the brain and cause symptoms).

PET scans rely on radioactive chemicals that are linked to some other compound of interest and injected into a person's bloodstream. These radioactive compounds emit a particle called a "positron" that is converted into pictures.

Glucose (fluoro-deoxy glucose, or fdg) PET scans can detect distinct patterns of diminished brain metabolism compatible with Alzheimer disease and frontotemporal lobar dementia.

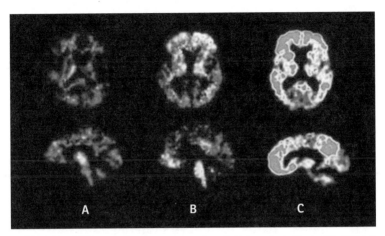

Amyloid-beta PET scans showing a range of amyloid deposits in the brains of those with normal cognition or with Alzheimer disease. **A** shows no evidence of amyloid deposits in the brain of someone with normal cognition. **B** shows some evidence of amyloid deposits in the brain of someone over age 70 with normal cognition. **C** shows significant amyloid deposition in the brain of someone with Alzheimer disease.

Amyloid PET scans show if the abnormal protein is located in the brain and, if so, where it is.

SPECT scans use radioactive particles called "photons." The images are less detailed than those produced by PET scans and are less expensive. SPECT scans are used to diagnose dementia with Lewy bodies and Parkinson disease dementia.

Q10. Why is the amyloid PET scan only helpful if the person is under age 70?

A10. After age 70, many people who are normal in their thinking have "positive" amyloid PET scans, meaning the scans show that they have beta-amyloid deposited in their brains. This is shown in the figure in *Q9*. It is not currently known whether all individuals over age 70 who have normal thinking but an abnormal amyloid PET scan will eventually develop Alzheimer disease.

Q11. If there is no blood test for Alzheimer disease, why was blood drawn when my husband was evaluated?

A11. Blood is drawn as part of the evaluation of dementia because a number of medical diseases can cause the symptoms of dementia. Among these are vitamin B12 deficiency and diseases of the thyroid, kidney, liver, and adrenal glands. Blood tests can detect these and other potential causes of dementia that can be treated. Some uncommon causes of dementia have specific blood tests that the doctor might order if they are suspected. Blood levels of certain medications are available and can determine if the dosage is too high and possibly causing cognitive impairment. Scientists are working to develop blood tests to help diagnose Alzheimer disease but so far they have not proven accurate enough.

Q12. Are there specific tests to diagnose the other 99 forms of dementia?

A12. Each of the other forms or causes of dementia has a distinct clinical picture that is different from Alzheimer disease. As a result, making the correct diagnosis depends on:

- The information the doctor elicits about symptoms and concerns. A disorder other than Alzheimer disease is suspected when the symptoms develop suddenly, have not worsened over time, developed when a new medication was started, or have been present for only several months.

- Findings on the physical and mental status exam. A disorder other than Alzheimer disease is suspected if there is weakness, sensation loss, unsteadiness, persistent drowsiness, or depression when the person is first evaluated.

- The results of laboratory tests. Test results can suggest a disease other than Alzheimer disease.

Everyone with possible dementia should have a thorough assessment because a potentially treatable cause of their symptoms might be detected.

Q13. Does mild cognitive impairment (MCI) fit under the dementia umbrella? What is the likelihood that a person with MCI will develop a dementia?

A13. MCI is best thought of as a condition between normal aging and dementia. The evaluation for MCI and dementia are the same, but in MCI:

- The person may have a decline in only one aspect of thinking.

- The decline in that one aspect of thinking is not as severe as the decline seen in dementia but is greater than seen in normal aging.

- The person may not be experiencing any decline in everyday functioning.

The technical definition of MCI requires that the person has a decline of 1.5 to 2 standard deviations on a test of cognitive performance compared to people who are similar in age and education. This indicates a 30% to 65% likelihood that the decline is meaningful compared to the 95% likelihood that is required for a diagnosis of dementia.

About 10% of people with MCI develop dementia each year after the diagnosis of MCI is made. This means that about 50% of people with a diagnosis of MCI will meet criteria for dementia by the fifth year after diagnosis. In those people with MCI who develop dementia, Alzheimer disease is often the underlying disease, but MCI can also be the earliest symptom of other illnesses causing dementia, including vascular dementia, dementia with Lewy bodies, and Parkinson disease dementia.

About 25% of people who meet criteria for MCI return to normal a year later, but these individuals are still at increased risk of developing dementia in the long run.

Q14. I took my wife to our local memory evaluation center and they recommended neuropsychological testing. It seems expensive. Should we go through with it?

A14. There are 2 levels of cognitive testing. Primary care physicians, neurologists, geriatricians, and psychiatrists administer short cognitive tests that take 5 to 10 minutes. These tests assess abilities in memory, executive function, perception, and language (see Q8).

Neuropsychologists are trained to administer batteries of tests that are much more detailed and comprehensive. The results of this testing are very helpful in certain circumstances but are often not necessary for making an accurate diagnosis, assessing the severity of the dementia, or making treatment recommendations. Because this testing is expensive and time consuming, I recommend it only in the circumstances mentioned below.

The tests administered by neuropsychologists are particularly helpful in distinguishing normal aging from the earliest signs of mild cognitive impairment (MCI) and dementia (*see Q2*). In-depth testing is helpful when a person has, or is suspected of having, depression, since certain tests can help distinguish a mood disorder from a cognitive disorder—or may suggest that both are present. Neuropsychological tests are also helpful in identifying which aspects of cognition are relatively unaffected and which are more severely impaired. This determination can help identify a specific cause of dementia.

Neuropsychological testing is particularly helpful in unusual situations, for example when someone is young, having trouble at work, or experiencing symptoms whose cause is unknown. Even if it is unclear whether someone is experiencing the earliest symptoms of MCI or dementia, neuropsychological tests can provide baseline data to which subsequent testing can be compared.

---

*Q15. My mother has been diagnosed by her primary
care doctor as having vascular dementia. Does it really
matter what the cause of dementia is?*

A15. Vascular dementia is the most difficult cause of dementia to diagnose accurately. Even when dementia experts diagnose vascular dementia, they are wrong 25% to 50% of the time, if autopsy is used as the standard. Most often the correct diagnosis is Alzheimer disease. However, in the past decade it has become clear that the relationship between Alzheimer disease and vascular dementia is complicated. They occur together more than would be expected by chance. This has led many experts to conclude that brain vascular disease likely contributes to the development of Alzheimer disease.

Vascular dementia is most accurately diagnosed when there are signs of prior stroke on the neurological examination *and* evidence of one or more strokes on a brain MRI or CT scan. Some doctors, however, make the diagnosis when there is evidence on a brain MRI of changes compatible with brain vascular disease without evidence of stroke. I believe that anyone with a diagnosis of probable vascular dementia should be carefully assessed for the presence of Alzheimer disease and that the treatments for Alzheimer disease be considered, because both diseases might be present.

I do believe it is important to obtain as accurate a diagnosis as possible. If the diagnosis is vascular dementia and future strokes can be prevented, then the person will not decline. Some causes of dementia, including normal pressure hydrocephalus (NPH) (*see Q92*) and chronic subdural hematoma, can be surgically treated. An accurate diagnosis also determines whether anti–Alzheimer disease medications or anti–Lewy body dementia medications are prescribed. Obtaining an accurate diagnosis helps predict the future development of new symptoms, information that is important for care planning.

Q16. What is Lewy body dementia?
How is it diagnosed and treated?

A16. Dementia with Lewy bodies (DLB) was identified as a common cause of dementia in the 1980s. The Lewy body is the microscopic pathological hallmark of Parkinson disease, and in Parkinson disease it is generally seen in a very specific area of the brain called the "substantia nigra," so named because it normally looks black.

DLB was first identified when a group of doctors in England noticed that some patients they had diagnosed with Alzheimer disease when living had Lewy bodies (*see the figure in Q9*) in the outer layer of their brain, the cortex, at autopsy. When these doctors looked at the medical records of these patients, they realized that visual hallucinations and mild parkinsonism (meaning Parkinson disease–like symptoms) were present in almost all the patients, usually very early in the disease.

DLB is diagnosed when dementia and Parkinson-like symptoms develop *within one y*ear of each another. About 85% of people with DLB experience visual hallucinations. The dopamine transporter SPECT scan (DAT scan) (*see Q9*) is abnormal in dementia with Lewy bodies.

Q17. Does Parkinson disease cause dementia?

A17. Experts argued about this question before there were good treatments for Parkinson disease, because it was difficult to distinguish between the slowing down and soft voice characteristic of Parkinson disease and changes in thinking characteristic of dementia. Because they are so effective, the drug treatments for Parkinson disease have dramatically improved quality of life, diminished the movement symptoms, and extended life span, but they also revealed that half or more of people with the illness will develop declining cognition at some point in the disease. This is referred to as "Parkinson disease dementia (PDD)." Many people with Parkinson disease do not develop cognitive decline, even after years of physical symptoms. Some people with Parkinson disease also develop Alzheimer disease, because both diseases become common as people age. People with the dementia of Parkinson disease have difficulty accessing what they know and early problems with visual perception. Many people with Parkinson disease are able to come up with correct answers or perform activities correctly, if given time. This is not dementia, it is slowing.

Parkinson disease dementia is diagnosed when a person has had Parkinson disease for *more than* one year before the symptoms of dementia begin. People with Parkinson disease dementia usually have impairments in memory, executive function, and perception but not in language or praxis (*see Q8 for a discussion of these symptoms*). The dopamine transporter SPECT scan (DAT scan) is abnormal in both Parkinson disease and Parkinson disease dementia (*see Q9*).

> Mental and physical slowing may be caused by Parkinson disease, but this is not the same thing as dementia. Many people with Parkinson disease are able to come up with the correct answer or do something correctly if they are given time. This is not dementia but *slowing*.

Q18. What is frontotemporal dementia?
What are tauopathies?

A18. Frontotemporal dementia (FTD), also called "frontotemporal lobar dementia (FTLD)," refers to a group of diseases with different clinical symptoms but with similar microscopic abnormalities. Distinctive abnormalities are found on the glucose (fdg) PET scan and MRI (*see the figure in Q9*).

The name of the disease derives from the primary location of the brain abnormalities. FTD starts in the frontal lobes, temporal lobes, or both. By contrast, Alzheimer disease originates in deeper structures of the brain and abnormalities are seen in the parietal lobes on PET scans.

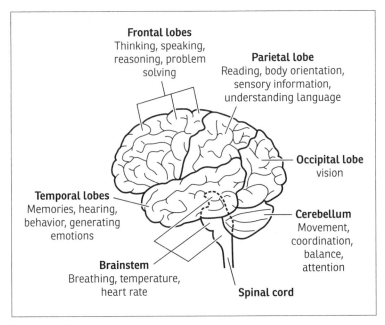

Frontal lobes
Thinking, speaking, reasoning, problem solving

Parietal lobe
Reading, body orientation, sensory information, understanding language

Occipital lobe
vision

Temporal lobes
Memories, hearing, behavior, generating emotions

Cerebellum
Movement, coordination, balance, attention

Brainstem
Breathing, temperature, heart rate

Spinal cord

Lobes of the brain.

In the early stages of FTD the symptoms can often be divided into two categories. The *language variant* of FTD begins with impairments in the expression or comprehension of spoken language. In some forms of this variant, people are aware of their speaking difficulties and become frustrated, but in other forms they are unaware of their deficits.

The *behavioral variant* of FTD begins in the frontal lobes, the part of the brain that controls executive function, the aspects of thinking that oversee, supervise, and coordinate cognitive function (*see Q8 and Q18*). Intact executive function underlies mental flexibility and the understanding of social cues. Given the complexity and subtlety of executive function, it is not surprising that the symptoms can be difficult to detect at the beginning of the disease. Early manifestations of impaired executive function include apathy (difficulty initiating activity), inflexibility in situations that are taxing, socially inappropriate language or behavior, inappropriate spending, and difficulty meeting the demands of work, house upkeep, or paying taxes.

Memory is often intact in both variants during the first several years of the disease. This is an example of why memory loss is not required for making a diagnosis of dementia. Over time, though, people usually develop symptoms of both variants.

At present, about one-third of people with FTD have a genetic cause for their disease, but in the majority of people with FTD, no cause can be found.

At autopsy, FTD is characterized microscopically by tau protein deposition, loss of cells in the frontal and/or temporal lobes, and a bubbly pattern referred to as "granulovacuolar degeneration (GVD)" (*see the figure in Q7*). Some people with FTD also have Pick bodies (another microscopic abnormality which was first described by Dr. Alzheimer in 1911) and/or the abnormal protein TDP-43.

The term "tauopathy" is used to refer to any disease characterized by tau protein deposits seen under the microscope. In addition to FTD, one of these diseases is *progressive supranuclear palsy (PSP)*. People with this disease become stiff, have a backwards curved neck, move and think slowly, and lose the ability to voluntarily move their eyes. *Cortical basal ganglionic degeneration (CBD)* is another tauopathy. People with CBD are unable to recognize or use their arm or leg even though there is no evidence of weakness in that limb.

Q19. What is amyloid angiopathy? My father was diagnosed last year at age 51 and can no longer live by himself.

A19. *Cerebral amyloid angiopathy* (CAA) is a disease in which repeated strokes lead to dementia. It is caused by the deposition of the beta-amyloid protein along the walls of blood vessels in the brain. These deposits weaken the blood vessel walls and cause them to burst. The resulting bleeding within the brain is called a "hemorrhagic stroke."

CAA usually develops in midlife. Because they have experienced multiple strokes, people with CAA often become unable to care for themselves within several years.

Some people with more classic Alzheimer disease also have amyloid deposition along the smaller blood vessels in their brain. This might be one reason that Alzheimer disease and vascular dementia occur together more often than they should occur by chance.

At present there is no treatment for the disease. Keeping blood pressure low does not prevent the bleeding into the brain. Whether amyloid-lowering drugs will lower the risk of strokes has not yet been determined.

Q20. What is CTE?

A20. It has been known for more than 100 years that boxers are at increased risk of developing dementia. More than 60 years ago, brain autopsy studies of boxers revealed the presence of neurofibrillary tangles, one of the abnormalities seen in Alzheimer disease. In the past this dementia was called "dementia pugilistica" because of its association with boxing, but now it is called "chronic traumatic encephalopathy (CTE)."

CTE has received a lot of attention in recent years because it appears to be associated with repeated head trauma in athletes playing American football, ice hockey, and soccer. There is increasing evidence that individuals who have experienced repeated concussions and head trauma in other settings are also at increased risk. At autopsy, which now is the only way to confirm the diagnosis, deposits of the tau protein are found deep within the folds of the brain.

The relationship between these disorders and Alzheimer disease is not clear and is being studied intensively. Both CTE and Alzheimer disease are characterized by tau deposits, but the deposits are usually located in different places in the brain. People who die from Alzheimer disease usually also have neuritic plaques at autopsy. Memory impairment is usually the first symptom of Alzheimer disease but may not be in CTE.

Since many fewer people with CTE have been studied, it is difficult to make general statements about the disease at present. It is thought that the earliest symptoms of CTE are related to damage directly or indirectly involving the frontal lobes. Early symptoms are thought to include irritability, apathy, changes in personality, and impaired judgement.

Q21. Can alcohol or other drugs cause dementia?

A21. Many prescribed medications, over-the-counter medications, and legal and illicit substances can cause cognitive impairment. Prolonged, heavy alcohol use can directly impair brain cell function, but not all experts agree that it can cause permanent cognitive impairment on its own. Part of the difficulty in demonstrating cause is that heavy users of alcohol are also at increased risk of developing cognitive decline due to a nutritional deficiency and at high risk of sustaining a traumatic brain injury from a fall, being hit in the head, or having an automobile accident.

Long-term heavy marijuana use has been shown to result in cognitive impairment in some people. Sedating drugs such as opiates (including morphine, heroin, and codeine) can suppress breathing and lead to the death of brain cells from lack of oxygen. Sedating benzodiazepine drugs (including Valium, Xanax, and Ativan) can directly cause an inability to form new memories that is often reversible if the drugs are discontinued. High doses of benzodiazepines can suppress breathing and lead to a lack of oxygen that kills brain cells and results in dementia. Volatile organic compounds that are inhaled (including gasoline, spray paint, and solvents) can permanently impair brain cell function and cause cognitive decline, slurred speech, and poor balance.

Many prescribed and over-the-counter medications can impair memory formation and cause cognitive impairment. They include antihistamines such as Benadryl (diphenhydramine), as well as drugs for the following conditions: high blood pressure, heart rhythm disturbances, pain (including opiates and NSAIDs such as ibuprofen and naproxen), bacterial infections (including penicillin and ciprofloxacin), viral infections, depression, psychotic mental illnesses, muscle stiffness and rigidity, respiratory conditions, insomnia, seizures, and Parkinson disease. Steroids can cause thinking impairment. Some cancer chemotherapy drugs may cause cognitive difficulty (referred to as "chemo brain"), but this has not been well established. In addition, interactions among these and other drugs may cause cognitive decline.

Most of these drugs cause *delirium*, an often reversible disorder that is characterized by cognitive decline and inability to pay attention (*see Q70*). If the offending drug can be stopped, recovery is common, but if there is another underlying cause of dementia, the decline in cognition will not fully resolve.

Many prescribed and over-the-counter medications impair memory formation and cause cognitive impairment. These medication side effects may resolve if the offending medication is stopped.

Q22. Should we try to arrange a brain autopsy for my mother who is diagnosed with Lewy body dementia?

A22. Brain autopsies may be available for people enrolled in research studies that follow participants over time, but otherwise they are difficult to obtain. Most Alzheimer Disease Research Centers do not need additional autopsy material. Many communities do not have an expert in neuropathology, the subspecialty that would perform such an examination. Most research programs have limited ability to provide the service, and there is a significant cost associated with obtaining an autopsy.

It is true, though, that autopsy is the final and most accurate way to identify the cause or causes of dementia. As a doctor I have found autopsy to be a good way to continue my education. I have incorrectly attributed dementia to the wrong cause and learned from my error. Autopsies often reveal that multiple causes are present in very old individuals.

An autopsy might improve doctors' ability to make the correct diagnosis in other family members in the future. This may be important for people in subsequent generations, since it could become the basis for recommending a preventive treatment that has to be taken for many years before the disease is likely to start.

3

What Causes Dementia? What Causes Alzheimer Disease?

Q23. Is dementia an accelerated process of aging?

A23. In my opinion there are many reasons to distinguish between usual aging and Alzheimer disease, but from a scientific perspective, the distinction has not yet been completely proven.

We know that there are many people who live into their 90s and even past age 100 who do not have symptoms of dementia. We also know that as a group, the brains of people with dementia are different from the brains of people who do not have dementia at every age. Furthermore, the mild declines in word retrieval and speed of performance that accompany healthy aging are different from the impaired ability to learn new information and organize daily life that are characteristic of most people with mild cognitive impairment (MCI) and early Alzheimer disease.

Everyone over the age of 85 has tau deposits in their brain, and many people who have tested as cognitively normal within a year or two of death have other pathological abnormalities, such as neuritic plaques, small strokes, Lewy bodies, and scarring in the hippocampus. Some people cite these findings as evidence in favor of the idea that dementia develops from an "aging" process.

In the past several years, scientists have learned that aging is associated with an increasing likelihood of developing gene mutations that can cause cancer. I do not think we would consider this "normal," but it is certainly an aging-associated process. The same might be true for the protein abnormalities that underlie progressive neurodegenerative dementias such as Alzheimer disease, Lewy body dementia, Parkinson disease, Parkinson disease dementia, and the tauopathies. That is, as we age, the likelihood increases that abnormal forms of certain brain proteins develop. If these abnormal proteins then slowly spread throughout the brain, dementia results. This is only a hypothesis, but it would help explain the strong association between aging and the risk of developing dementia.

Q24. Is Alzheimer disease hereditary?

A24. The answer to this question turns out to be complex.

People who inherit an abnormality in 1 of 3 genes, called "PS1," "PS2," and "APP" (amyloid precursor protein), develop Alzheimer disease, almost always before the age of 65. These genes are very rare in the population and account for 1% to 2% of all cases of Alzheimer disease.

50% to 60% of the risk of developing the common late-onset form of Alzheimer disease is related to more than 25 genes. Here's where the genetics gets very complex and is not fully understood.

One of these genes, called the "*APOE* gene," contributes about half of this genetic risk. The other half is contributed by the remaining 25 or so genes.

The *APOE* gene has 3 forms, labeled 2, 3, and 4. Each is considered a "normal" gene variant. Since we inherit 1 copy of the *APOE* gene from each parent, we can have 1 of 6 possible combinations of the *APOE* gene. This means each of us is either 2/2, 2/3, 2/4, 3/3, 3/4, or 4/4.

The 4 form of the gene (labeled "*APOE4*" or "*APOE ε4*") increases the risk of developing Alzheimer disease, such that people who are 2/4 or 3/4 have a 2.5 to 3 times *greater risk* of developing Alzheimer disease than people who do not have a 4 form of the *APOE* gene. A person who inherits 2 copies of the 4 gene (4/4) has about a 12 times greater risk of developing Alzheimer disease than someone who has no copies of the 4 form of the gene. There is good evidence that the 2 form of the gene actually *lowers* the risk of developing Alzheimer disease.

Surprisingly, the *APOE4* gene is not 100% determinative. A number of people have been identified who are very old, have 2 copies of the *APOE4* gene, and do not have Alzheimer disease.

If two-thirds or so of the risk of developing Alzheimer disease is genetic, then roughly one-third is nongenetic or environmental. It is a mistake, then, to think that what happens in life is either "genetic" *or* "environmental." This used to be referred to as the "nature vs. nurture" or "gene vs. environment" debate. It turns out that most common diseases do not follow this either-or model—they are caused by *interactions between* genetic risk factors and environmental risk factors. This is a whole new understanding of illness. Much research is needed to explain how such interactions cause disease.

Q25. Should I get genetic testing if my mother has Alzheimer disease?

A25. If a parent, brother, or sister (all referred to as "first-degree relatives") has clinically diagnosed Alzheimer disease, then your risk of developing Alzheimer disease is 2.5 times to 3 times more likely than someone whose parents and siblings (brothers and sisters) did not develop Alzheimer disease. It is easy to obtain genetic testing through over-the-counter gene testing kits such as 23andMe. However, before you do so you should understand what these tests can and cannot tell you. The best source of information about genetic testing is a trained genetic counselor, but most people either do not have access to such an expert or do not think they need to seek out their advice. In the next few paragraphs I will try to simplify what is a very complex issue.

As discussed in *Q24*, the *APOE* gene is the strongest genetic factor affecting the risk of developing the common form of Alzheimer. Over-the-counter gene-testing kits test for this gene.

In thinking about the value of these tests, it is important to know that the risk that any individual will develop Alzheimer disease by age 80 is, conservatively speaking, about 20%. This risk rises to about 35% if the person has 1 copy of the *APOE4* gene. If a person has only *APOE2 or APOE3* copies of the *APOE* gene, then that person's risk of developing Alzheimer disease by age 80 decreases to about 15%. Thus, undergoing genetic testing for the *APOE* gene tells most people whether their risk of developing Alzheimer disease *by age 80* is 15% or 35%. For the small number of people who have 2 copies of the *APOE4* gene—about 5% of the population—the risk of developing dementia by age 80 is significantly higher.

To me, a 15% risk is significant and the difference between 15% and 35% is small. This has led me to conclude that *every* adult has a meaningful risk of developing Alzheimer disease by age 80, because the average life expectancy in the United States is 80 years for women and almost 79 years for men.

My own conclusion is that genetic testing for Alzheimer disease can tell people who have a family member with onset before age 60 whether they have inherited a copy of the *PS1, PS2,* or *APP* gene mutations and are at very high risk of developing Alzheimer disease (*see Q24*). For everyone else, the test kits give very little information beyond what we know already from population risk statistics: Everyone is at risk of developing Alzheimer disease if they live long enough, since many people with no *APOE4* gene develop the disease. If knowing your genetic risk information would lead you to live your life differently, then you should probably consider doing so, no matter what the gene test shows.

I recognize that many people believe that genetic information would make a difference to them. I have no problem with making such tests and information available to them as long as they understand what the results can and cannot tell them. Not surprisingly, research shows that many people who get tested are hoping they will find out they are not at increased risk. My advice is that you should get tested only if you want to know if your risk is 15% or 35% at age 80, if you want to know whether you are one of the small percentage of people who have 2 copies of the *APOE4* gene and are at much higher risk, or if you have family members with the disease who developed symptoms before age 60 or 65, in which case the possibility is increased that you have inherited one of the abnormal dominant *PS1*, *PS2*, or *APP* genes.

People who are concerned about a family history of fronto-temporal dementia or Huntington disease should contact a genetic counselor if they are considering being tested.

Q26. Why do researchers think that the beta-amyloid protein or the tau protein causes Alzheimer disease? How do medications for treating Alzheimer disease target these proteins?

A26. As described in Q7, Alzheimer disease is characterized by 2 microscopic brain abnormalities: *neuritic plaques*, which consist of the protein beta-amyloid surrounded by pieces of dead nerve cells, and *neurofibrillary tangles*, which consist of twisted fibers made up of the protein tau.

There are many lines of evidence supporting the hypotheses that these abnormal proteins, either singly or in combination, are the cause of, or directly contribute to, the death of brain cells in Alzheimer disease. However, since this connection has not been proven, it is still possible that plaques and tangles are only markers for some other disease process that has yet to be discovered.

Evidence has been mounting that the beta-amyloid protein starts accumulating in the brain 15 to 20 years before the first symptoms of Alzheimer disease. Most studies find that tau is deposited in the brain closer to when symptoms start.

Neuritic Plaques

The amyloid protein seen in the neuritic plaque (*see the figure in Q7*) is derived from a larger protein called the "amyloid precursor protein (APP)." APP is a normal constituent of the cell membrane of every neuron. When brain neurons die, the APP is broken down into fragments by enzymes. These fragments are then removed from the brain through the spinal fluid that bathes the brain, through the bloodstream, and through another system, called the "lymphatic system" (*see Q29*).

However, some people are prone to form a fragment of the amyloid precursor protein called "A beta$_{42}$" (because it is 42 amino acids long). A beta$_{42}$ is too large to be removed from the brain, and therefore accumulates. The amyloid theory of Alzheimer disease is based on the finding that this A beta$_{42}$ is toxic and kills other brain neurons. The dead cells then release more A beta$_{42}$, which kills more brain cells. This ever-increasing cascade of cell death is the cause of dementia, according to this theory.

This hypothesis might be thought of as a problem in "garbage disposal." If the A beta$_{42}$ could be removed, the theory goes, then the whole cycle of cell death causing more A beta$_{42}$ causing more cell death could be halted.

Many of the drugs in development to treat Alzheimer disease have targeted this "amyloid cascade." Drugs have been designed to *remove* the toxic A beta$_{42}$ protein, to *decrease the production* of the A beta$_{42}$ protein, or to *increase the production* of the "nontoxic" form of A beta (A beta$_{40}$). So far, none of these drugs has slowed or stopped the progress of Alzheimer disease in humans, although some have been successful in removing A beta$_{42}$ protein from the brains of people with Alzheimer disease.

People with Down syndrome all develop the plaques and tangles characteristic of Alzheimer disease by the time they reach their 40s and are at higher risk for developing the dementia of Alzheimer disease by their 60s. The increased risk is likely related to the cause of Down syndrome, which is an extra copy of chromosome 21, on which is located the gene that makes the amyloid precursor protein (see Q24). As a result of their extra chromosome 21, people with Down syndrome have 3 copies of the APP gene rather than 2, and they produce 50% more of the amyloid protein.

Neurofibrillary Tangles

The second abnormality in Alzheimer disease, the neurofibrillary tangle (see the figure in Q7), is made up of abnormal forms of the tau protein. Normally this protein is part of skeleton-like structures within cells which help the cell keep its shape. In Alzheimer disease, these structures become abnormal and lead to cell death. The amount of tau in the brain correlates with the severity of Alzheimer disease, so tau, too, has been a target of drug development. One drug designed to remove tau from the brain has failed to slow the disease. Other drugs are being developed to remove or prevent the deposition of the tau protein.

Several explanations have been proposed for the failure of the anti-amyloid and anti-tau approaches. One is that the drugs have been started too late in the disease process—remember, the A beta$_{42}$ protein is being deposited 15 to 20 years before the first symptoms. A second potential reason is that both the A beta$_{42}$ protein and the tau protein need to be removed. A third possibility is that some other process initiates the formation of plaques and/or tangles, and this other process must be identified and targeted if a treatment is to work. A final possibility is that alternative approaches are needed to better remove these abnormal proteins.

Q27. Are there environmental causes of Alzheimer disease?

A27. Yes. Nongenetic and environmental factors appear to contribute 30% to 50% of the risk of developing Alzheimer disease. Potentially changeable risk factors that have been identified are high blood pressure in midlife and less early-life education. Some studies have found increased rates of Alzheimer disease in people who have experienced depression in the past, engaged in less physical activity, were less engaged socially, are overweight, have hearing impairment, have elevated blood lipids, and have had a prior head injury.

As discussed in *Q80* and *Q81*, environmental risk factors and genetic risk factors interact. Many genes establish a vulnerability, but disease emerges only if an environmental trigger is present. This radical rethinking of how diseases are caused is just beginning to affect how doctors treat and prevent disease.

Q28. What do you think about the theory that Alzheimer disease may be "germ" related?

A28. Several lines of scientific evidence support this possibility. One is that the amyloid precursor protein (APP) (*see* *Q24 and Q26*), a protein that is in the cell membrane of every neuron in the brain, functions as an anti-infection protein. If this is accurate, then some infectious agent might cause the release of APP and start the cascade that leads to the deposition of the amyloid (A beta$_{42}$) that is characteristic of Alzheimer disease (*see Q26*).

Another possible link to infection is indirect evidence that a herpes virus infection earlier in life is linked, many years later, to the formation of the plaque lesions of Alzheimer disease. A third possible link to an "infectious" process involves *prions*, a name derived by combining letters from the words pr*oteinaceous, infectious,* and *particle* ("ons" means "particle"). Prions cause Creutzfeldt-Jakob disease (CJD) and the related "mad cow disease" (officially called "variant Creutzfeldt-Jakob disease," or "vCJD"), both of which cause a rapidly progressive dementia. The prion protein is a normal protein that can transform into an abnormal form that has the amazing ability to make copies of itself. These copies continue to multiply, enter nearby cells, and cause cell death. Because vCJD and some forms of CJD are acquired from eaten, injected, or implanted tissues that contain abnormal prions, they are considered infectious, and in that way act like "germs."

Prions do not cause Alzheimer disease, Lewy body dementia, Parkinson disease dementia, or frontotemporal lobar dementia, but the mechanism by which prions spread through the body and brain might be similar to the mechanism by which the abnormal protein characteristic of each of these diseases spreads within the brain.

***Q29. I know that disrupted sleep can be a symptom
of Alzheimer disease, but I have heard that disturbed
sleep might be a cause of Alzheimer disease. Is there
any truth to that idea?***

A29. Disrupted sleep has long been known to be associated with
Alzheimer disease (*see Q78*). Recent studies suggest that the
beta amyloid protein is removed from the brain by the lymphatic system, a system of connected tubules that drain fluid
and immune cells. In mice, the lymphatic removal of amyloid
protein breakdown products from the brain occurs at night—
raising the possibility that in humans, disrupted sleep decreases the removal of these breakdown products and the tau
protein, and thereby leads to Alzheimer disease. Conversely,
Alzheimer disease might directly damage the areas of the brain
that control sleep and thereby decrease the lymphatic system's
ability to remove amyloid.

4

What Steps Can I Take to Lower My Risk of Alzheimer Disease and Dementia?

Q30. Are there any steps I can take to lower my risk of developing Alzheimer disease? My mother was diagnosed with Alzheimer disease and both of her parents had dementia.

A30. The identification of what can be done to *prevent* Alzheimer disease is in its infancy. Such studies are very difficult to carry out because they require having thousands of people do a certain activity, follow a specific diet, take a specific medication, or follow a specific lifestyle for many years. There is, however, strong indirect evidence that the following actions can *lessen* risk:

- engaging in **moderate physical activity** for 30 minutes a day, 5 days a week

- ensuring **maximal treatment of high blood pressure and blood lipid abnormalities, especially in midlife**

- eating a **heart-healthy diet** that is low in animal fat and high in fruits, vegetables, and natural omega-3 fatty acids

- engaging in **enjoyable mental and social activities**

Many of these have been proven to decrease stroke, heart attack, and vascular disease. This further supports the link between brain vascular disease and Alzheimer disease.

Q31. Do computer games, crossword puzzles, Sudoku, or cognitive training prevent Alzheimer disease?

A31. There is no evidence that such activities prevent the development of Alzheimer disease or dementia. A few studies have found that people can improve their performance on these specific activities with repeated practice, and that this benefit lasts for as long as 10 years. This training may lessen the cognitive changes that accompany *normal* aging.

Q32. Are there diets, vitamins, or other foods that can prevent dementia?

A32. Diets or diseases that cause deficiencies of vitamins B1, B6, and B12 can cause cognitive impairment. A well-balanced diet is enough to ensure adequate intake of B1 and B6, but some people develop an inability to absorb vitamin B12, and low levels of vitamin B12 can cause dementia. For that reason, anyone developing memory or cognitive decline should be tested for B12 deficiency, even though it is an uncommon cause of dementia.

There is some evidence that a "Mediterranean diet," a diet in which red meat intake is low, vegetables, fruits, and nuts are eaten regularly, and olive oil replaces other fats, can lessen the cognitive declines that accompany normal aging. This does not mean that this diet lowers the risk of Alzheimer disease, however.

In my opinion there is no convincing evidence that antioxidant foods, omega-3 fatty acids, nuts, a ketogenic diet, a Mediterranean diet, supplements formulated to enhance memory, or a low-salt diet prevent Alzheimer disease. Some of these may have other health benefits, however. I also know of no evidence that ginkgo biloba, turmeric, jellyfish protein, or coconut oil prevent Alzheimer disease.

Some studies have shown that regular, modest intake of red wine is associated with a lower risk of dementia. However, a recent analysis of all studies that have examined potential health benefits of alcohol found no such association.

Q33. Does Alzheimer disease vary in frequency by country? Rural/urban populations? Gender?

A33. By and large, Alzheimer disease has been found to occur with the same frequency at any given age throughout the world. There are a few exceptions, but these tend to be in groups or places in which it is unusual to live to a late age. However, most studies comparing different populations rely on diagnoses made by researchers or doctors, not on autopsy-confirmed diagnoses. For this reason, I consider the final answer to your first 2 questions to be unknown.

Most experts now agree that women are at greater risk of developing Alzheimer disease than men, even after correcting for the fact that women have a longer life expectancy than men. The reason or reasons for this are not known.

Q34. What influence does diabetes have on developing Alzheimer disease?

A34. People with diabetes are at higher risk of developing dementia, but the specific cause or causes of this increase are not clear. One possibility is that diabetes increases the risk of developing vascular dementia. Another is that diabetes directly causes dysfunction and death of brain cells. So far, there is no evidence that better control of diabetes lowers the risk of developing dementia.

Q35. Do you really think it will be possible to prevent Alzheimer disease when it seems that everyone in their 90s has evidence of the disease in their brains? Doesn't that imply that we will all get the disease if we live long enough?

A35. Yes, I do think it will be possible to prevent Alzheimer disease, or at least to significantly lower people's risk for developing it. One strategy that could accomplish this is to delay its onset for so long that most people will die from some other cause before they develop Alzheimer disease.

Several pieces of data lead me to be optimistic. First is the finding that the abnormal proteins characteristic of Alzheimer disease are present in the brain years before the first symptoms of dementia appear. This suggests that the body has some innate ability to fight off the disease, but that these protective mechanisms become overwhelmed over time. It also raises the possibility that very early recognition of amyloid or tau deposition could indicate when to start treatment and thereby prevent symptoms from ever developing.

Second, several well-designed studies have found that the rate of onset of dementia ("incidence rate" is the technical term) has declined in the past decade. A combination of the following is thought to account for this decline: better treatment of high blood pressure and high blood lipids; declining rates of stroke; greater participation in exercise; lowered intake of red meat and other foods that increase the risk for arteriosclerosis; and the prevention of heart attacks and strokes by using stents and medications.

A third reason for optimism is that Alzheimer disease probably has multiple, interacting environmental and genetic causes. This raises the possibility that a combination of the following approaches might further lower the risk of developing the disease: additional small improvements in exercise, diet, and lowering of cardiovascular risk factors; the development of treatments that decrease the deposition of abnormal proteins in the brain; the stimulation of new connections among brain nerve cells and pathways; and the formation of new brain cells in areas vulnerable to cell death related to Alzheimer disease.

Finally, the identification of genetic risk factors raises the possibility that we will be able to target preventive treatments to those who are genetically at increased risk of Alzheimer disease, and, thus, improve the likelihood of an individual's benefiting from a preventive intervention.

Q36. Why hasn't more progress been made in coming up with a cure for Alzheimer disease?

A36. Several very challenging mysteries related to Alzheimer disease are yet to be solved. First, even though there is strong evidence that abnormal protein deposition begins 15 to 20 years before the first symptoms appear, it is not known what *starts* this process. Identifying this trigger would greatly aid the search for effective treatments.

Second, it is not yet clear how to detect these very early brain changes. This will be crucial, since any preventative or "curative" drug or drugs will need to be started when the brain degeneration first begins, if not before.

Third, most parts of the brain are not able to make new brain cells. As a result, even if the disease could be stopped in its tracks, replacement brain cells would not form on their own in most brain areas. One exception is the hippocampus, in which new brain cells do develop throughout life. Treatments that begin before the disease moves out of the hippocampus might allow new cells to form and replace those that have died. It will still be a challenge for these new cells to connect correctly to cells in other areas of the brain.

5

What Treatments Are Available?

Q37. Can people with Alzheimer disease learn new things? *My husband was diagnosed about a year ago and can remember some things (not everything, but neither can I) that happened days ago.*

A37. The answer is "definitely yes" and "it depends on the cause of their dementia."

People with mild cognitive impairment (MCI) and mild Alzheimer disease are able to learn new information, although not as well as they once did. As MCI evolves into Alzheimer disease or another cause of dementia, this ability to learn and retain new information becomes increasingly impaired.

There are **several different types of memory.** Alzheimer disease initially impairs the memory system that is responsible for the **learning of facts**—for example, remembering what you ate for breakfast this morning. Information that has strong emotional significance, whether positive or negative, is more likely to be recalled.

The ability to **learn new tasks**, called "procedural memory" or "motor memory," is relatively preserved in people with early and mid-stage Alzheimer disease. This ability may even be present into later-stage disease. As a result, people with Alzheimer disease can learn *to do* new activities. The ability to learn a new task improves with repetition, as it does in everyone. The learning of a new task is also enhanced by starting small and building up to more complex sequences, and by minimizing the pressure to learn.

Because there are multiple types of memory, and because each type of memory involves a somewhat distinct set of brain structures, different causes of dementia lead to impairments in different types of memory or to the development of impairments in a different order. For example, the dementia of Parkinson disease initially impairs the ability to *access* memory. As a result, people with the dementia of Parkinson disease are slow to answer questions and to perform requested actions but retain the ability to learn new facts into the moderate stages of dementia. In the early stages of frontotemporal dementia (FTD), memory for new facts is often normal. Generalizations about memory cannot be made about vascular dementia because the location of the strokes in any particular person determines what structures and systems are impaired.

Q38. What do you think about music therapy?

A38. Many people with dementia respond to music in a very positive way, especially to music they knew and enjoyed earlier in their lives. Examples include popular songs from their youth and younger adulthood, hymns, anthems, and the alma mater of their high school or college.

Music has a number of elements to it. These include rhythm, tune, words, and tempo. To some extent, each involves a different brain area. This may explain why some people who have lost the ability to speak can still sing, or why someone who has trouble dressing can still play an instrument like the piano. Also contributing to the high value that most people and cultures place on music is its engagement of and association with particular emotions (*see Q37*). These emotional linkages probably strengthen the memory for familiar music.

Music is an effective and important form of treatment for many people with dementia. The joy it brings them attests to its power. If the person with dementia is unable to identify favorite songs or types of music (hymns, classical, rock 'n' roll, or hip hop), family members or friends might be able to do so.

> Music engages many people with dementia. It provides pleasure and helps them maintain connections with their past and with others.

Q39. My wife used to love the symphony but recently she has been very reluctant to go. The last time we went she demanded that we leave early. Isn't it important for her to stay active?

A39. Yes, helping your wife stay active and engaged is important, but she should be the guide and have the final say in what she wants to do. Taking her to the symphony makes sense, since this is an activity she has always enjoyed, but her behavior might be telling you it is now overwhelming her. She may be uncomfortable sitting for a long period or being with a large number of people. If so, perhaps she would be more comfortable if you took her to a shorter musical event in a smaller setting. Perhaps she would enjoy listening to music from a playlist you put together for her, from an online music site, or on the radio.

I have what I jokingly refer to as "The Three-Strike Rule." If you try something 3 times and your wife resists each time, it is probably overwhelming for her.

> If you try something 3 times and each time it leads to distress or resistance, that likely is a sign that the activity is overwhelming for the person with dementia. If possible, avoid or minimize the frequency of that stimulus.

Q40. Does exercise slow down the progression of Alzheimer disease and other dementias?

A40. This is a controversial issue about which there is significant disagreement. Some studies have shown that people with mild cognitive impairment (MCI) and dementia have a slower progression of their symptoms if they participate in a physical exercise program, but others have not. When the studies are considered as a whole, the evidence is not yet convincing, in my opinion.

Physical exercise, including walking, has many benefits, including improving the quality of life for many people with dementia. Studies of exercise in middle-aged and older people have shown that it lowers the risk of future stroke and heart attack. Importantly, Tai Chi has been found to decrease the risk of falling.

My conclusion is that everyone should be offered the opportunity to engage in a daily physical activity program that is safe for them. People may choose not to become involved or to drop out. Clearly, it is inappropriate to force people to become more active. Finding out what people did earlier in life might identify activities they would be interested in doing now.

Some diseases that cause dementia impair balance, strength, and judgement. Before starting a new exercise program, people should be assessed to determine what they are capable of doing safely and what they are no longer able to do. Even if exercise does not slow the progression of dementia, its other benefits support the conclusion that everyone with dementia should be encouraged to exercise regularly.

> **Everyone should be offered a daily physical activity program that is safe for them.**

Q41. What do you think of day care for people with dementia? It is expensive and I am not sure it is worth the money.

A41. I am a strong supporter of day care because it is a way for people with dementia to remain stimulated, active, and supported. At the same time, it is a way for family caregivers to get a break from their caregiving role.

If cost is an issue, ask what the minimum attendance is (how many days a week), and ask if there is a sliding-scale fee schedule based on your income or assets. Some programs have access to state funds, donations, grants, or "scholarships" for individuals who need financial assistance.

Q42. How will I know when to place my wife in a long-term care facility? Is it inevitable?

A42. Placement is not an inevitability for people with dementia, but there are many people with dementia whose care needs are greater than their family can provide. At any one time only about 30% of people with dementia live in assisted living or a skilled nursing facility, but for people whose dementia progresses to a severe stage, more than 75% live in a long-term care setting.

Most of the time there is no single trigger that leads to placement. Rather, an accumulation of issues, such as the need for physical care beyond the capability of the caregiver, ill health in the caregiver, behavioral symptoms that are beyond the family's ability to manage, and multiple, chronic medical issues, together make it dangerous or impossible for the person to stay at home. My clinical experience is that families often wait until there is no alternative.

Possible placement should be discussed openly with family members. If people have different views of the needs of the ill person, you may need to get information from your wife's primary care doctor or nurse, from a dementia care specialist, or from an occupational therapist who has done a home assessment. Everyone involved in the decision-making process should know what the ill person can and cannot do, what the person's medical needs are, what the daily support needs are, and whether the current situation is safe. If you are the primary care provider you should feel free to openly discuss your emotional well-being, financial issues, and health issues. If disagreements can't be resolved, try to find a third party such as a social worker, counselor, or dementia care expert who can guide the discussion.

Some people go to long-term care immediately after a hospitalization, but a majority move directly from their home. Research has shown that those who move to a long-term care facility are older and have more severe dementia, more behavioral and psychiatric symptoms, and fewer available family members to provide care.

Guilt about placing a person out of the home is common among caregivers. However, one study I carried out found that many people with dementia became more active when they moved to long-term care. Many caregivers felt that they and the person with dementia had benefited. A common reason cited by the caregivers was that they were no longer providing nursing care and so were able to return to the role of a loving family member.

One benefit of attending a support group is finding out that many others are struggling with the issue of placing a loved one. This may not lessen your guilt or make the decision any easier, but it can help to know that you are not alone in dealing with a disease that forces people to be moved to a place where they can receive 24-hour care. If you are struggling with the decision, it may be helpful to talk with friends who have faced the same decision or to discuss it with clergy, a social worker, or your doctor.

Q43. How do I find a good nursing home?

A43. If you know people who have previously placed a relative in long-term care, ask them if they are happy with that facility and why or why not. Ask members of your support group, the local Alzheimer support agency, your doctor, health practitioner, or clergy about facilities they know that deliver excellent care. Medicare publishes ratings of skilled care facilities, but these ratings primarily look at how facilities comply with regulations—an important issue but not one that is necessarily tied directly to the quality of care.

Visit several facilities. Is the person you talk with knowledgeable about the needs of people with dementia? Ask them what dementia-specific programs they offer and how they know what is best for an individual resident. Ask what kind of staff training they require and offer. Observe how the staff interacts with people who have cognitive problems. Are they engaged with them and treating them as people? Good facilities should not smell of urine.

Make sure you have adequate information about financial issues. What are the person's remaining assets? Do they have long-term health care insurance? Will they need to spend down their assets to become eligible for Medicaid? Can they and you afford the facility that you choose?

Q44. I was surprised to learn that Medicare doesn't pay for nursing home care. Why is that?

A44. Medicare was designed to be an insurance program for acute care needs. Since all dementias are chronic illnesses,

When looking for a long-term care facility,
- Ask others who have placed a loved one about their experiences.
- Visit several facilities and ask what dementia-specific programs they offer.
- Ask how they will know what is best for an individual resident.
- Observe how the staff interacts with people who have cognitive problems.

long-term care services for dementia are not covered by Medicare. However, people with dementia may be hospitalized for acute problems and may need rehabilitation or brief, ongoing care such as intravenous antibiotics. These services are covered by Medicare.

Some years ago, Congress passed a bill establishing a program for long-term health care insurance, but opposition was so widespread that the program was rescinded the next year.

Q45. My husband has been living on a nursing home unit that has locked doors because he had wandered away from home on several occasions. How do I know when it's safe to remove him from this locked-door facility?

A45. Some people with dementia are at increased risk of bad outcomes from accidently or purposefully leaving where they live. They would be unable to find their way back and risk exposure to dangerous situations. Others have a very low or no risk of leaving, or live in a setting where going out the door leads to a safe enclosure. A general goal for all of us is to move freely about unless we are at a high risk of a bad outcome, such as a fall. At a minimum, this means that people who are at high risk of harm if they do go outside on their own should be able to move about freely *within* a facility.

If a person's risk of wandering off is very low or nonexistent, then living on a unit that has locked doors seems overly restrictive to me, but some facilities offer only a locked-door environment. If your husband does not need the protection provided by a locked door, I suggest considering whether the benefits of where your husband is living now outweigh any potential benefits of his moving. If not, then moving him is certainly reasonable. However, if the locked door is primarily a concern of yours and not his, then moving him may be adding an unnecessary trauma.

The idea that some units have locked doors is distressing to many people. I believe they are sometimes a necessity, because we are obligated to protect people who are unable to protect themselves. Some people are so driven to leave that reasonable attempts to secure an unlocked exit are doomed to fail. For them, I know of no less restrictive environment than one in which the exit doors are locked.

Q46. Should I reintroduce my father's dog, which we had to remove from his house because she was upsetting him?

A46. Many people with dementia respond just as positively to animals as do people without dementia. Most professionals have seen people with dementia who have been withdrawn and minimally responsive to human interaction become active and animated when dogs or cats are present. This is sometimes referred to as "pet therapy," and it certainly deserves to be described as such. Several clinical trials of pet therapy for people with dementia have demonstrated a variety of positive benefits.

It sounds like you made the difficult decision to remove your father's dog because you concluded that the risks of harm to the dog and upset to your father significantly outweighed the pleasure your father would have experienced. That certainly makes sense to me. However, I agree with you that it is worth trying to reintroduce his dog and see what happens. You might try having your father and the dog together several times to see if problems arise. If being around the dog still makes your father upset or exposes the dog to harm, then they should not be together.

One of the most important things I have learned about decisions like this is that you can only figure out the best answer by *trial and error*. There are many circumstances in which we don't know what the right decision is and can only find out what is best by trying different approaches.

Q47. Do the anti-dementia drugs like Razadyne, Exelon, Aricept, and Namenda work?

A47. The evidence is clear that these medications work better than a sugar pill (placebo), but there is disagreement among experts about how much of a benefit they provide, how long they should be prescribed, whether they should be prescribed in very high dosages, and whether they are worth the cost.

About one-third of people with Alzheimer disease and Parkinson disease dementia experience a measurable improvement in thinking and daily function when treated with the anticholinesterase medications Razadyne (galantamine), Exelon (rivastigmine), or Aricept (donepezil). As I look at the evidence, which is contained in the package insert that pharmacists distribute with every prescribed bottle of pills, this benefit is the equivalent of about 6 months of disease progression. This means that if people start the medication in September and have an average response, they improve to the level of cognition and function they had the prior March. This describes an average response—some people will have no benefit, some will have an average response, and some will benefit more than the average.

Interestingly, for the first 3 weeks of treatment there is a "placebo response," meaning that people who are randomized in research studies to take a non-active pill have the same benefit as people who take the active medication. By 6 weeks, though, this placebo response disappears and those on the active medication have improved cognitively while those on placebo have not.

The anticholinesterase drugs can cause a number of side effects. These include nausea, vomiting, diarrhea, slowed heart rate, falls, nightmares, and poor appetite.

If the drug is stopped after several months, cognition returns to where it would have been had the medication never been taken. This demonstrates that the medication has not slowed or reversed the underlying disease process that destroys brain cells and their connections to other cells. Rather, Razadyne, Exelon, and Aricept work by increasing the availability of a chemical, called "acetylcholine," that is deficient. This is similar to what insulin does in diabetes and L-dopa does in Parkinson disease.

Memantine (Namenda) works differently from the anticholinesterase medications. It decreases the overstimulation of nerve cells that occurs when cells are injured. When prescribed alone it is not as effective in treating Alzheimer disease as the anticholinesterase drugs, but it is better than a placebo pill.

One study has shown that the combination of memantine plus an anticholinesterase medication is better than a cholinesterase inhibitor alone (Aricept was used in the trial, but I presume the same would be true of Exelon and Razadyne).

Q48. How long should a person stay on anti-dementia medications?

A48. Many people who ask this question report that they see no benefit within several months of starting one of these medications or that any benefit they saw has disappeared. Unfortunately, all the studies that have attempted to answer this challenging question are significantly flawed.

The best study, in my opinion, examined people who had remained on Aricept and Namenda for 2 years and determined whether those staying on the medications for a third year were better than those who stopped the drugs. Everyone in the study declined in both thinking (cognition) and daily function during the third year, but those on Aricept declined less.

I interpret this result to mean that people who have remained on Exelon, Aricept, or Razadyne for a long time *may* still be benefiting very modestly. However, since most people do not stay on any anti-dementia medication for 2 years, there is no way to know how applicable the results are to people who have taken the medication for a shorter time. I know this is a frustrating answer, but it is the best information we have. Since the benefit is so modest, anyone experiencing significant side effects should probably stop the medication. If there are no side effects, then the decision to continue or stop anti-dementia medication depends on how one weighs the desirability of a small benefit.

Q49. What are your thoughts about medication treatment for depression in people with Alzheimer disease? What about other treatments?

A49. About 20% of people with Alzheimer disease have symptoms of clinical depression. Symptoms suggesting depression include either agitation or withdrawal, weight loss, disrupted sleep, and hopelessness (*see Q80*). The rate of depression is higher in people with vascular dementia and people with dementia due to Parkinson disease. The likelihood of having symptoms of depression at any time during the course of Alzheimer disease is 30% to 40%.

Only about half of studies of antidepressant medications in people who have both dementia and clinical depression have shown benefit. Likewise, studies of exercise alone have shown mixed results.

My opinion is that for a person with dementia who also has symptoms of mild or moderate depression, the first focus should be on making sure there are no medical illnesses or medications that might be causing depression. Also, the person should be offered and encouraged to engage in activities that they would enjoy and be able to participate in. Some people with mild cognitive impairment (MCI) and mild or moderate dementia are able to talk about their feelings and should be encouraged to do so. Although this has not been shown in studies to be beneficial, it seems a reasonable thing to try as long as the person agrees and is not upset by the conversation. Some people with dementia have symptoms of more severe depression. In my opinion it is reasonable to offer such individuals an antidepressant medication, even though the evidence supporting their effectiveness is weak.

Q50. Should people with mild cognitive impairment (MCI) take Aricept and Namenda?

A50. Neither drug is FDA approved for the treatment of MCI, and the evidence for any benefit is very weak. However, I know that some doctors do prescribe these medications for people with MCI, their reasoning being that every potentially beneficial treatment should be tried. While I would not do so, I think this is reasonable as long as the person with MCI understands the lack of evidence of benefit and accepts the risk of side effects.

Q51. What do you think about preparations like ginkgo, coconut oil, turmeric, and jellyfish protein?

A51. Of these, ginkgo is the best studied and has not shown any benefit as a treatment for Alzheimer disease. The other 3—coconut oil, turmeric, and jellyfish protein—have not been adequately studied, but the little evidence I have reviewed does not suggest they are beneficial, for either the prevention or the treatment of Alzheimer disease. Coconut oil may elevate blood lipids, which is potentially harmful. I see no harm in trying these, since side effects are rare, but they can be expensive. On the other hand, I worry about raising hopes unrealistically. Benefit from any of these is very unlikely.

Q52. Why do antipsychotic drugs increase death in people with Alzheimer disease? Are they ever appropriate? What are alternative approaches to problematic behaviors?

A52. Antipsychotic drugs such as Seroquel (quetiapine), Abilify (aripiprazole), Haldol (haloperidol), and others have been greatly overprescribed for people with dementia. They have been used to treat sleep problems, pacing, wandering, complaining, and mild suspiciousness. There is no evidence that antipsychotic medications are effective in treating these issues and a great deal of evidence that these drugs cause many severe side effects. *All* drugs in this class have been shown to increase mortality rates in people with dementia between 60% and 100%. This increased death rate occurs within 12 weeks and persists for at least 1 year after treatment starts; it may continue as long as people are taking the drug.

This increase in mortality is likely due to multiple causes. People with dementia who take antipsychotic drugs are more likely to die from cardiovascular disease, infection, and, probably, fall-associated mortality.

In the rare circumstance in which these medications are necessary, they should be prescribed in the lowest effective dose, stopped if there is no benefit, reassessed after several months even if effective, and discontinued if at all possible.

A small percentage of people with dementia have physical agitation or delusional (untrue) beliefs that are causing them significant distress and interfering with their ability to enjoy life. Rarely, very agitated people with dementia cause harm to others. To address these issues, most expert clinicians agree that non-drug approaches should be tried before antipsychotic medication unless there is an acute emergency for which no treatment other than medication is available. The *first step* in addressing physical aggression and delusional beliefs is to determine if there are triggers that can be addressed. The triggers might be medical, emotional, neuropsychiatric (such as hallucinations or delusions), or environmental. There are often multiple possibilities, so it can take time to go through them. *Trial and error*, that is, seeing if something works and, if there is no benefit, going to the next possibility, is an important principle. If the solution were obvious it probably would already have been tried (*see Q46*).

Antipsychotic drugs are rarely necessary to treat symptoms of dementia, and they increase mortality rates in people with dementia between 60% and 100%. In the rare instance in which they are needed, they should be prescribed in the lowest effective dose, stopped if there is not significant benefit, reassessed after several months even if effective, and discontinued if at all possible.

Whenever there has been a sudden change in behavior or alertness it is imperative to consider whether a new medical event has occurred. It is also important to review whether any new medications have been added or medication dosages changed within the prior month, since these may trigger changes in function and behavior.

While the assessment for possible causes of physical agitation and delusional beliefs is underway, attempts should be made to involve the person in activities they are able to do and might enjoy. Although some individuals with dementia choose not to engage in activities, you are more likely to find something they would enjoy by trying to determine what activities they participated in prior to becoming ill.

When trying to engage people with dementia in activities, avoid pushing them to do things they are no longer able to do. Personal preference is of primary importance. Many people (with and without dementia) do not know if they would enjoy a new activity and will respond positively to encouragement and support.

---

*Q53. What is respite care? I understand that
some states pay for this as an alternative
to long-term care placement.*

A53. Respite care refers to services that provide 24-hour care for a brief period of time for people with dementia so their caregivers can have some time away from the caregiving role. For care providers who are at their wits' end and are feeling overwhelmed, respite care can be a life saver.

You are right that some states are providing a respite care

benefit in the hopes of delaying or preventing placement in long-term care, but it has not been proven that respite care delays moves to long-term care. Even so, I believe respite care is a wonderful temporary resource, and I strongly recommend it.

Q54. My mother has lost a pound or two a month for the past 6 months. Should I worry? Her appetite seems good when I am with her.

A54. In the general population, people over age 70 lose a pound or two per year on average. This is not explained by illness or lack of access to food.

If someone with dementia loses weight more quickly than this, a reason should be sought. For example, some people have always eaten between meals, so when snack foods are less available to them, they lose weight. Some older people have impaired taste and smell. If this diminishes the pleasure they get from food, they may eat less.

Many of the diseases that cause dementia impair chewing and swallowing in the more advanced stages of the disease. If people with dementia cough when drinking or choke on food or fluids, they may have a neurological impairment of the swallowing mechanism or be unable to coordinate the multiple actions that go into drinking, eating, and swallowing. Speech and language pathologists are experts in assessing swallowing and may be able to identify a cause and make recommendations that improve a person's ability to eat and take in calories.

In end-stage dementia some people seem to actively resist eating. When I examine such people, they usually have a strong suck reflex, something that is seen in newborns. One manifestation of this reflex is biting down on a spoon or other eating utensil that is put into the mouth. One sign of an impaired chewing and swallowing mechanism is the accumulation of food in the cheeks.

If no treatable cause of a swallowing disorder is found, several steps can be taken to improve calorie intake. These include serving foods the person has always liked, allowing people to finger-feed themselves, taking time (even 60 to 90 minutes) to feed those who are unable to feed themselves, providing small amounts of food throughout the day, pureeing food if the person cannot chew, and using thickened liquids, which are easier to swallow than thin liquids.

There is no evidence that feeding tubes prolong life or prevent aspiration (the introduction of food or secretions into the lungs) (*see Q91*). In my opinion, the decision to place a feeding tube is as much an ethical question as a medical issue (*see Q101*), and the substitute health care decision maker or family members should have the final say (usually the person with advanced dementia is no longer able to participate in the discussion).

Q55. Are people with Alzheimer disease eligible for the hospice benefit under Medicare? If so, what symptoms suggest that a person with dementia is appropriate for hospice care?

A55. Yes, people with dementia are eligible for hospice care and now make up a significant proportion of those who receive treatment under the Medicare hospice benefit. In the past there were specific hospice eligibility criteria applicable only to people with dementia, but now the standard is that a physician certifies that the person has less than 6 months to live. Hospice should be considered for people with dementia who have had more than one episode of pneumonia, who are losing weight in spite of appropriate efforts to feed them, and who are bedridden or unable to walk independently. Among the benefits that hospice provides are help with daily care needs, increased focus on comfort and pain management, support of the family, and helping loved ones prepare for the person's death. Most hospice care is provided in people's homes or in long-term care facilities, not at an inpatient hospice facility.

Q56. Do people die from Alzheimer disease?

A56. Pneumonia is the most common cause of death in people with dementia. Because all the diseases that cause progressive dementia eventually impair swallowing, people with advanced dementia from any cause are at high risk of aspiration, meaning that food, secretions from the mouth and nose, and contents of the stomach go into the lungs rather than down the esophagus (the swallowing tube that connects the mouth and the stomach) (*see Q91*). Aspiration is a common cause of pneumonia.

People with dementia are at high risk of falling and breaking a hip or other bone, of developing side effects from medications, and of developing delirium (*see Q70*). All of these shorten life expectancy in people with dementia.

Because the dementia is the direct cause of the swallowing impairment, and because the swallowing impairment leads to aspiration and pneumonia, the dementia is considered to be the initiating cause of death when a person with late-stage dementia dies from pneumonia. This is true for all diseases that cause progressive cognitive decline. Since Alzheimer disease is the most common cause of dementia, it is often stated that Alzheimer disease is the fifth or sixth most common cause of death in the United States.

6

What Suggestions Do You Have for Caregivers?

Q57. I heard you say that people with dementia can experience a positive quality of life, even when the disease is severe. I can't imagine that. In fact, I can't think of anything worse than knowing you have Alzheimer disease.

A57. I appreciate your raising this because others have made similar statements in my office, but rarely is the issue brought up in public. I will answer it both from my clinical experience and from a research perspective.

When I interact with people who have dementia, they often seem happy, engaged, and aware of what is going on. Of course, some people with dementia are sad, distressed, and not engaged. When I have conversations with people who are aware that they have dementia, many of them tell me that life seems the same; they might not be able to do everything they want, but when they are with family and friends, when they are engaged in activities they enjoy, or even when just sitting around, they say that, all in all, things are "OK" or "could be worse." I do not want to sugarcoat what it means to have dementia, and do not want to downplay the fact that not everyone is so positive. However, I have treated medically and psychiatrically ill people throughout my career and remain struck that people face adversity in many different ways. Many can recognize the negatives of their illness or situation and yet appreciate what they have had in the past and still have.

In my research on quality of life in people with dementia, several findings bear emphasizing. First, some people with dementia experience a positive quality of life throughout their disease, even when it is severe. Second, the main aspects of quality of life in people with dementia are a positive mood, enjoyment of activities, amount of social interaction, awareness of their past, and awareness of their surroundings. Third, many people simultaneously express negative and positive thoughts about their current situation. Finally, people experience and express similar types and ranges of emotion whether they have good health, dementia, or a major physical disability.

I have heard people make statements similar to the last sentence in your question about having a debilitating physical illness, undergoing an amputation, having a mental illness, becoming blind, and being diagnosed with a terminal disease.

Over my career I have observed a wide variation in how people respond to bad news. Some describe both negative and positive emotions while others report a predominance of one or the other. Having an opportunity to talk openly about the negative feelings seems to help many people feel better, but not everyone.

What has struck me the most when discussing "bad" medical news with people is that many people have the ability to adjust to very difficult circumstances. I do not believe this is denial or an inability to accept reality, and I recognize that it is more difficult for some people than others. The most common mistake I see in talking about the impact of bad medical news is to expect that everyone reacts the same. As a professional, my job is to help those who are suffering, but not everyone in difficult situations is suffering or needs professional help. This is as true for dementia as it is for other medical and psychiatric illnesses. I have learned that having dementia does not necessarily prevent you from being a wonderful grandparent, getting pleasure from visitors, enjoying being hugged, or watching others have a good time.

Q58. I have just been diagnosed with Alzheimer disease and am still working. Should I tell my boss? My family? My friends?

A58. This is a difficult question and one for which there is no single right answer. If you have a life partner, I do think you should tell that person and discuss your preferences about the future with them (*see Q59 about legal documents*). If you have children, I think you would want to tell them and also talk with them about the future. The same would be true for anyone who has a serious medical condition. Talking about your health with those close to you should give you a forum to talk about your fears and receive emotional support.

> In some circumstances, Social Security Disability Insurance benefits can be "fast tracked" if a person has dementia.

There are positives and negatives about informing work supervisors. The risks are that you will be asked to retire or be terminated and the difficulties this could cause for you. On the other hand, you may not be able to recognize whether your dementia is causing problems with your job now or in the future. If your illness is already causing problems at work, that could not only cause bad outcomes but lead to your termination and loss of disability benefits. Dementia is now recognized by Social Security as a cause of permanent disability. In some circumstances, Social Security Disability Insurance benefits can be "fast tracked" if a person has dementia. Over the years I have had many patients who did not know they had dementia and lost jobs as the result of declining job performance before they came for the evaluation.

If you have received a diagnosis of dementia and the disease is likely to progress, you should plan for the likelihood that someday you will not be able to make financial and health decisions for yourself.

Even though it was clear, in retrospect, that dementia had led to their job loss, they have generally been unsuccessful when they retroactively applied for disability.

As for as telling friends and acquaintances, I think it depends on how well you know them, how close you are with them, and whether you think something adverse is likely to happen. Today, most people know someone with dementia, often a parent or other relative. That should make them more understanding than people have been in the past. Not telling people out of shame does not make sense, but that does not mean that you have to tell everyone. Talking about this issue with your partner or someone you trust can help you decide whom to tell.

If you have received a diagnosis of dementia and the disease is likely to progress, you should plan for the likelihood that you will not be able to make financial and health decisions at some point. As I discuss in Q59, I think it best to immediately write a will and establish durable power of attorney documents both for health decisions and for financial decisions, if you haven't already done so. You should contact all financial institutions where you have accounts and find out what procedures they want you to follow to appoint someone to substitute for you in the future, because not all companies accept durable power of attorney documents. If you have a lawyer, you should discuss all these issues with that person.

Q59. What is the difference between designating a power of attorney and identifying a durable power of attorney? Can I change my will if I have dementia?

A59. These are complicated legal matters, and you should consult an attorney about the specifics of your situation.

In general, a power of attorney document appoints the person named in the document as someone who can substitute for you in the ways that you specify in the document. For example, you might appoint someone as your power of attorney if you will be traveling and know that a document to sell property must be signed while you are away. Importantly, you must be *competent* when you sign a power of attorney document. If you later become *incompetent*, meaning you are not able to make decisions for yourself, then the power of attorney document becomes void.

> Immediately after receiving a diagnosis of dementia, you should write a will and establish durable power of attorney documents for health and financial decisions, if you haven't already done so.

For this reason, all states and the District of Columbia have established documents titled "durable powers of attorney" or some similar label. The key word is "durable." This means that the document remains in force even if the person signing it becomes incompetent. These documents indicate whom you would want to substitute for you if you are declared incompetent. The specific mechanism by which a person is declared incompetent varies by jurisdiction.

Almost all jurisdictions separate the making of financial decisions (durable power of attorney for finances) from the making of health care decisions (durable power of attorney for health). Some states have added other categories. I believe strongly that all adults should legally identify a durable power of attorney because anyone can have an accident or develop a sudden, severe illness and become unable to make decisions for themselves. Unfortunately, most people do not have such documents. Receiving a diagnosis of dementia or a life-threatening condition such as cancer is often the trigger for doing so.

Many states also have established living wills or similar types of documents. In some states these documents are only applicable at the end of life, but many jurisdictions allow for people to express their health care wishes verbally to the person who will be making substituted decisions for them. In some jurisdictions, wishes about future care can be expressed in durable power of attorney documents.

There is a lot of variability about these issues, so it is important to be informed about the specific rules in the place where you live. You may be able to find this information online, from the attorney general's office of your state. Many health care facilities have information about these matters, as do local departments of aging. Family attorneys and estate attorneys are knowledgeable about these issues.

Wills dictate what is to happen to people's belongings, including money and property, when they die. If there is no will, the state will determine to whom and how the estate will be distributed. The opportunity to write a will was established by common law even before the United States became a country. The overriding principle reflected in legal precedent and legislation is that people should be able to distribute their estate however they want, even if others think their decisions are foolish. However, to write a will, people must know what a will is, must know, in general, what their assets are, must have some idea of how people commonly distribute their assets, and must express whom they want to inherit their belongings. People who have dementia and are able to do these things retain the capacity to write or change a will. However, people with progressively worsening dementia eventually lose the ability to know these things. This is why it is important to write a will if you receive a diagnosis of dementia and have not already done so.

Q60. Should a person stop driving when given a diagnosis of dementia?

A60. There is wide disagreement among knowledgeable experts on this issue. The answer also varies by state. Some states require that the motor vehicle bureau be notified when a diagnosis of dementia is made, while others do not allow physicians to break confidentiality and report the person's diagnosis.

All experts agree that people with moderate dementia due to any disease should not drive. By this stage of dementia, the likelihood of impaired judgement, perception, reaction time, and multitasking is high, and the risk of having an accident is significantly increased.

The disagreement about when to stop driving relates to people with mild dementia (recognizing that this is not a well-defined term). Studies have shown that accident rates are higher for people with mild dementia than for the average driver, but they are equivalent to the accident rates for teenage boys. Hence the dilemma.

Driving evaluations can be performed by some occupational therapists, and some states will provide driving evaluations if asked to by a person with dementia or by a family member, or if a professional reports that the person is possibly impaired.

If a person has had an accident after receiving a diagnosis of dementia they should stop driving, in my opinion, because one can never be sure that the dementia did not contribute. This is true even if the other driver is charged. Some professionals talk about the "grandchild test"—If you would not let a person drive your grandchildren, then they shouldn't be driving.

Q61. Our family has gone on cruises together once a year for the past 20 years. My husband was diagnosed with dementia of unclear cause 2 years ago, and I am wondering if we should continue this tradition. One of our sons says definitely not, while our other children agree with me that we should try it. What do you recommend?

A61. I am assuming from this question that your husband has always enjoyed going on the cruises. It also sounds like you would like to continue this tradition because you want to continue that source of pleasure for him and want to do something together as a family that has always been a source of fun for everyone.

The risks of going on a cruise with your husband include his getting lost in an unfamiliar place and the worry that would cause him and you. He might be less able to participate in shipboard and off-ship activities than he did in the past, and that, too, could be upsetting. He may need to have someone with him at all times to ensure his safety, but may resent this and not understand or accept the need.

There are many potential benefits of going on a cruise for your husband, you, and other family members. Your husband would be doing something familiar to him and something he has always enjoyed. For everyone in the family, going on the cruise would be a way to continue a family tradition that has long been special. For you, the cruise would be both a way to be with everyone in the family and a way for you, as the primary caregiver, to get away from caregiving when others are spending time with your husband.

If you went on a trip last year and there were no problems, the likelihood of major problems this year seems low. Since problems are still possible, you should ask your family how they would feel if problems did develop. If everyone accepts the low risk, then it is a risk worth taking.

If there were problems last year, then the likelihood of more difficulties this year is significant. I recommend discussing this openly with other family members.

Another possible approach is to take a short (2-day or 3-day) trip to a nearby hotel and see how that goes. If there are no problems, then a longer trip is likely to work out. Also, look into the availability of "dementia-friendly" cruises.

There is no way to predict whether a time will come when these trips are no longer possible. Every adult on the trip should be aware that your husband's dementia increases the risk of problems but does not make them inevitable. His safety and enjoyment are important. You should weigh both of these as you make your decision.

_____

Q62. My husband was diagnosed with Alzheimer disease about a year ago, but he continues to deny that he has anything wrong with his memory. He is able to drive and be left at home alone without any problems. Is there anything I can do to convince him that he has an illness that affects his memory? Is this denial?

_____

A62. More than one-third of people who have been diagnosed with Alzheimer disease are unaware of their difficulties or deny that they have problems when told of their diagnosis. An even higher percentage of people with Alzheimer disease will say things like, "Of course I have memory trouble. So does everyone my age." This is also evidence of unawareness.

In my opinion, this unawareness is usually a symptom of Alzheimer disease (*see Q94*). One reason for concluding this is that rates of unawareness are much lower in people who have vascular dementia or Huntington disease of the same severity. Even if I am wrong and this unawareness or denial is the result of an inability to "accept" the diagnosis, the bottom line is that the person either is unable to know or does not want to know. In either case, trying to "convince" him is not appropriate and can be upsetting to him.

Unfortunately, this unawareness can lead to problems if he should not drive, go out alone, be home by himself, pay bills, babysit, or take medications on his own.

I recommend that you always remind your husband that the diagnosis was made by his doctor. You could say, "Don't forget, Dr. Smith is the one who made the diagnosis." That way, if he disagrees, you can say, "Well, we are scheduled to see Dr. Smith in a few weeks. You need to tell him directly that you disagree." If there is something he should not be doing because it is dangerous you can add, "In the meantime, I don't think you should [*whatever the activity is, such as* go walking by yourself] until Dr. Smith gives the go-ahead."

Q63. How do I start a conversation with my wife, who has early-stage dementia, about getting additional support when she eventually needs more care?

A63. The answer depends on whether your wife is aware of her diagnosis and can appreciate that she has a problem. If she is able to recognize that she has dementia or a memory problem, then I suggest you have a general discussion about future plans. A good place to start is either establishing durable power of attorney documents and writing a will, if you and she have not already done so, or reviewing these documents, if you already have them. This discussion can provide an entrée into talking about and planning for a variety of possible scenarios for both of you in the future.

Use her response to guide how much detail you can go into. If she is becoming restless or upset, then back off a little. In general, I recommend trying to acknowledge her being upset ("I know this is hard to talk about. It is for me, too."), but if that further upsets her, then stop and restart the conversation another day. If she is able to talk about these issues, it may be helpful to discuss them as possible situations ("What if I get sick or am not able to help you as much as I need to?"). If her response is, "Oh, that will never happen," it is fine to say, "I hope not, but what should we plan to do if I can't give you the help you need?"

Such conversations are difficult for most people. Dementia can render some people unable to participate because of impaired reasoning capacity, because they become upset easily, or because they lack insight.

However, they still may be able to discuss these issues in a general way. You might try stating your preference for what you would like and then ask her what she would do. For example, "If I got really sick and needed more help than you could give, I would want [*whatever you would want, such as* to be cared for by home health care workers in our house]. How about you?"

Unfortunately, some people are not able to discuss these issues even when their dementia is mild. If you have had prior discussions about these issues, consider using those conversations as a guide to her preferences.

Q64. My 10-year-old daughter has asked several times why her grandfather, who has been diagnosed with Alzheimer disease, has changed. Should I discuss his diagnosis? What is she likely to understand?

A64. I do think you should talk with her and use her responses to guide you in deciding how much detail to provide. At a minimum, explain that what she has noticed is caused by a sickness. I suggest emphasizing that he loves her and that the family still loves him. Highlight the things they enjoy doing together. If she asks about the sickness, it is reasonable to tell her the name of the disease. There are several books written about Alzheimer disease for children and teens. She might want to read one alone and ask questions, or she might want to read it with you.

Q65. My 78-year-old father has cared for my mother for almost 3 years. I have suggested several times that he attend a support group, but he always replies that he doesn't need it. Is there anything I can say to him to convince him?

A65. I believe that support groups are a wonderful resource. I have always encouraged the caregivers I interact with to consider going to one. Support groups are a great source of information about community resources and potential solutions to challenging problems. They are also a source of emotional support from people who are facing similar challenges.

That said, support groups are not for everyone. Some caregivers are doing well and don't need more support or information. Other caregivers are too "private" for the experience that support groups offer. If your father seems to be doing well, I don't think you should try to convince him to go to a group.

On the other hand, if he seems demoralized, tired, angry, or overwhelmed, I suggest you gently share these observations with him and tell him that there are many sources of support available. Among them are family members, friends, clergy, counseling services, and support groups.

If he seems to be struggling emotionally I also recommend telling him that you are concerned about both your mother and him, and that his getting help will be good for both of them. If he is worried about the cost, find out if there is a charge; most support groups are free. You could offer to attend the group with him to test it out. If he continues to resist getting help and he seems to be doing worse, you might ask if he would consider respite care or long-term care for your mother.

Q66. My mother has always been a cheerful person and has done well as a caregiver for my father for several years. Recently, though, she has seemed sad and depressed. She talks much less on the phone, doesn't seem to want to see my children, and cries at the drop of a hat. I told her I was concerned that she was depressed, but she passed it off as "just part of being a caregiver." What do you think?

A66. Although being a caregiver doubles or triples the risk of feeling demoralized, the majority of caregivers never develop clinical depression. The fact that your mother seems "changed" from her usual self does suggest that she is experiencing clinical depression; her diminished energy, avoidance of usually enjoyed activities, and frequent crying further support this.

If a person with dementia can carry a phone, their primary caregivers should put their own phone number and that of other emergency contacts in "ICE" (In Case of Emergency), under "favorites," and in the phone's address book under "wife," "son," "daughter," or "friend."

I suggest telling your mother several things. First, tell her that you see her as a changed person and that this is *not* a usual outcome of being a caregiver. Tell her that she has certain symptoms (listed in the previous paragraph) that suggest she has clinical depression. Also tell her that you are only recommending that she be evaluated, and that, if you are wrong, then you will be relieved. Finally, tell her that there is strong evidence that depression responds to treatment and that research has shown that when depression in a caregiver improves, the mood and behavior of the person with dementia also improve.

***Q67. Since this is anonymous, I will tell you that I have
yelled at my husband twice in the past month. He has
dementia and I know it's wrong, but it happened so
quickly that I couldn't control it. I would never hit him,
but I feel so guilty. Do you think this means that I
should place him in a nursing home?***

A67. Guilt and frustration are very commonly experienced by caregivers of chronically ill people, particularly caregivers of people with dementia. Guilt may be a sign that you are overwhelmed, so you should ask yourself whether you need more help in the house, a brief vacation, or the help offered by a support group (*see Q53*).

I am guessing that you are not in a support group or, if you are, that you haven't mentioned that you yelled at your husband. If you had, you would likely have found that almost everyone in the group had done the same thing on occasion. And, like you, everyone would have expressed regret about it.

Frequent losses of temper suggest that a caregiver is overwhelmed, but occasional episodes are so common that I consider them normal. Finding an outlet for your frustration such as talking with friends, joining a support group, or discussing the matter with clergy can help, as can taking time away from caregiving. If the problem continues, consider talking with a counselor. If these steps don't help, you should think about alternative living situations.

Q68. How do you support a caregiver long distance?

A68. Only about half of family members live close to a loved one who has been diagnosed with Alzheimer disease. In most circumstances, when there is a partner living with the person or there are family members nearby, they shoulder most of the caregiving responsibilities. I think this is important for out-of-town family members to keep in mind, because it is often difficult to tell from a distance exactly what the issues are.

An important first step for people living out of town is to acknowledge that those living close by are most likely to know about the day-to-day issues, both positive and negative. Realize that both the person with the disease and those providing care need support. I suggest that you check in by phone regularly. I think phone is better than text or email, because it is more personal and you can detect some things by hearing that you cannot in writing. If you do check in regularly, be sensitive to the possibility that the caregiver might feel that you are checking up on them. If this might be the case, reassure the caregiver that you want to be kept in the loop and want to help, but that you are not questioning their ability. If you are concerned that the caregiver is overwhelmed or no longer able to provide what is needed, then you should try to visit in person to assess the situation.

I believe strongly that the more facts people have, the more likely they are to be able to figure out what needs to be done. Ask the caregiver to tell you about the results of visits to the doctor and other professionals after each contact. Recognize that many caregivers who are "on-site" or close by believe they are most knowledgeable about the situation. This may well be true. Ask about their observations and opinions.

Visit as often as possible to see for yourself how things are going and to assess what is needed. If possible, provide some caregiving yourself and give the person providing most of the support some time off. Make sure that your visit is not adding to the caregiver's responsibilities.

Encourage the local caregivers to utilize available agencies and supports. Be sensitive to the possibility that they might see this as admitting defeat. Recognizing that regular caregivers may be reluctant to use extra help is important, because you might be able to convince them that getting this help is best for both the ill person and the caregiver. If the caregiver believes that no one can do as good a job as they do, empathize with their dilemma—they may be correct, but getting extra help might still help things go more smoothly. You may need to repeat your offer to relieve the caregiver more than once.

Q69. How do I find good people to help me at home?

A69. Getting help at home can prolong a person's ability to remain in their own home, a goal of almost all people with dementia and caregivers. Some caregivers need help with tasks such as bathing, dressing. or moving a bedbound person, while others need help with meal preparation, cleaning the house, or respite from caregiving. All of these are valid reasons to get help at home. Of course, there are many others.

Many agencies provide this kind of help. If you know someone else who has obtained help, ask them. They may be able to recommend an agency or a specific person who has helped them, or refer you to someone who knows what or who is available. If you are in a support group, ask people if they can recommend someone or some agency. A social worker may know of an agency that pays special attention to the needs of people with dementia.

Make sure the agency is bonded. This means that the agency has reviewed the credentials of the people they hired and has made arrangements for you to be reimbursed if theft or financial abuse occurs.

If you are unhappy with the person, let the agency know. Tell them directly what your concerns are, and ask the agency if there is someone else who can better meet your needs. If you hired a person directly and are unhappy with their services, you can terminate them and try to find a more suitable person, but keep in mind it might take a while to find a replacement.

> If you are looking for help at home, ask people who have already had this kind of help. They may be able to recommend individuals, agencies, or referral services.

Q70. My father has dementia and is scheduled to go into the hospital next week for a hip replacement. Is there anything I need to worry about because he has dementia?

A70. Dementia increases the risk that he will develop delirium as a complication of the anesthesia, surgery, or postoperative medical care. *Delirium* is characterized by a sudden worsening of *cognition* (thinking) and an altered level of *alertness* (people are either drowsy or hyperalert). Delirium prolongs hospital stays, interferes with recovery and rehabilitation, increases the cost of care, and increases the risk of dying in the next year. Importantly, delirium can be prevented if the following steps are taken:

- the person is frequently reminded where they are and why they are there ("You had hip replacement surgery yesterday and will be in the hospital for 2 or 3 days."),

- careful attention is paid to the person's fluid status by the medical team,

- medications are carefully monitored and the person is on the lowest doses possible,

- lighting is adequate during the day and minimized at night,

- unnecessary noise is eliminated,

- the person is encouraged to walk as soon and as much as is medically safe, and

- physical and occupational therapy are started as soon as possible.

I recommend having a family member or paid sitter with your father *24 hours a day.* This person should remind him, as frequently as he needs, where he is and why he is there, keeping in mind that he may not remember what he has been told after just a few minutes. This person can also answer his questions, keep him stimulated when he is awake, and call staff if there is a problem.

Q71. My mother, who was diagnosed with Alzheimer disease several years ago, has started accusing me of stealing money from her. This really hurts, because she lives with us and I am her primary caregiver. I know these ideas probably come from the disease, but it still hurts me when she says it.

A71. This is a common and distressing occurrence. You know it isn't true but others who hear the accusation may not. If that is the case, discreetly let them know that this is a symptom of her disease.

If someone else is being accused, do your best to find out whether the accusation is true. Unfortunately, there are people who take advantage of those who are ill and dependent.

The person making the accusations may be misplacing a purse or wallet and assuming that someone has taken it. If that is the case, ask if you can help her look for it. If this helps, keep an extra purse or wallet in her room. Some people are reassured if they have a few dollars readily available. If having some money reassures her, show her the wallet with the money and give her an out, such as, "I can understand how upset you were when you couldn't find your wallet."

One frequently effective approach is to distract and reassure the person. If you tell her you will look into it but ask her if she could, for now, help you with a chore or tell you what happened earlier in the day, she may become engaged and forget about her accusations, at least for a while.

Avoid antipsychotic medications if at all possible (*see Q52*). Suspiciousness and accusations should not be treated with medication unless they place the person or someone else at meaningful risk of harm.

Q72. My brother has been diagnosed with Alzheimer disease and now has a lot of trouble coming up with words and names. Should I help him, or is it better for him to stimulate his memory by trying to find the words he wants to say on his own?

A72. When we do physical exercise, we generally think that the harder people work, the more benefit they get. However, we know that when people have been physically injured and are unable to do an activity, they benefit more if we provide them with the help they need to function and participate actively. For example, if a person has had a stroke and is very weak on one side, we provide the support needed to stand and walk—a cane or walker, for example—and design a rehabilitation program that seeks to strengthen their weak muscles.

A similar principle should be applied to helping people with dementia and other diseases that impair thinking. Many people with dementia who have word-finding problems are frustrated by their difficulty in retrieving the words they want to say. This frustration makes it even harder for them to retrieve the word they are searching for. I conclude from this that most people with a language impairment caused by dementia (*see Q8*) do better when they are given the word they appear to be searching for. This enables them to continue the conversation, which is their goal. If you are not sure what word your brother is trying to say, you can give him several words to choose from.

Occasionally, people become more frustrated or angry if you try to supply them with the word they are searching for. If that happens repeatedly, stop giving them suggestions. You can ask them what their preference is, but they often are unable to understand that question or express a wish.

Some people with the language disorders of Alzheimer disease or frontotemporal dementia (FTD) do not recognize their impairments or are unable to use words to clarify what they want to say. People with this kind of aphasia are sometimes not able to recognize that they are having a problem communicating.

Most people with a dementia-caused language impairment do better when they are given the word they appear to be searching for.

Some people with language problems are able to understand nonverbal cues, that is, communication through visual or tactile information. For example, if you are asking someone to walk to the dining table and move your body in that direction, they are more likely to comprehend your request than if you only use words. Gently touching their elbow and directing them towards the dining room is a way of nonverbally communicating the same information.

Q73. Is there anything I can do when my wife refuses to take her medications?

A73. It is important to make sure that she (and each of us) is only taking medications that are necessary and potentially beneficial. Reducing the number of pills by eliminating unnecessary medications, by giving medications as few times per day as possible, and by maximizing the amount of medication in a single pill can sometimes help with this problem.

Ask your wife if there is a reason she doesn't want to take the medication. Does it taste bad? If she is taking pills, does it hurt to swallow them? Does she feel that her situation is hopeless and that taking medication will not help? If she is able to express a reason, is there something that can be addressed to make the situation better for her? Some medications have longer-acting formulations that are equally effective and would decrease the number of times that she is presented with pills. Ask her if she would prefer a liquid. Find out if a patch is available and, if so, ask her if that would be more acceptable. Determine if she is more comfortable taking a few pills at a time over 15 to 20 minutes.

Some people are more accepting of care at one time of the day rather than another. If such a person is refusing medications, ask her health practitioner if you can give the medication at the time of day when she is more likely to cooperate. There are medications for which a dose can be safely skipped once in a while, but this is uncommon. Ask her doctor or nurse what to do if a dose is skipped.

It is important to find out whether the person who is refusing medication has the ability to make a choice based on the risks and benefits of the medications. This determination depends on an assessment of competency by a professional. One reason to appoint a durable power of attorney for health is that the designated person can make such judgements for someone who has become, and has been declared, incompetent to make such decisions. Just because a person with dementia refuses a medication, medical test, or medical intervention does not mean that they lack the competency to make decisions. *If* the person is competent and able to weigh risks and benefits, we should honor their wish.

People have different opinions about surreptitiously putting crushed pills in food like applesauce or dissolving them in a liquid if a person is refusing to take medications. I believe it is appropriate to do so *if* the person has lost the competency to make medical decisions and *if* the individual who is their substitute decision maker agrees that this approach is acceptable. I recognize that this ignores a person's freedom to choose, but if they have been declared incompetent to make medical decisions, they are not able to make reasoned choices.

Q74. I am concerned that my husband will wander away from home. I want him to be safe, but I also want him to have as much independence as possible. What technology can I use to make things safer?

A74. An "old" technology, a bracelet with a person's name, phone numbers for emergency contacts, and diagnosis, is worth looking into. If he regularly carries a wallet, put a card with emergency contact information in one or several places in it.

Cell phones offer features that can make a person safer. Many phones have health apps or "ICE" (In Case of Emergency) settings that can be accessed even if the phone is locked. Put your phone number and that of other emergency contacts in "favorites" so someone can contact you. Also list contact information in the phone's contacts' list under "wife," "son," "daughter," and "friend" to identify who should be called in case of an emergency.

Your husband may be able to remember how to use his cell phone even if he is becoming forgetful. Make it as simple as possible for him to call you and have him practice doing this. People with Alzheimer disease retain the ability to learn new tasks for a long time, even if they have trouble remembering recent events. This is why your husband may be able to learn how to use a cell phone even if he hasn't had one before, or learn a new way to get in touch with you using a phone he has had for a while (*see Q37*).

The Health App has an emergency contact, or "ICE" (In Case of Emergency), button.

Call your husband regularly so your name and number will be listed in "recent calls," which is another place a stranger might look for emergency contacts. If you have labeled your contact information as both "wife" and "ICE," these labels will appear on the recent calls list.

There are apps that can help you locate or follow your husband. They vary by phone manufacturer and carrier. They have names like "Find My Friends" and "Find My Phone." The Health App has an emergency contact, or "ICE" (In Case of Emergency), button. Locator chips that are made to help find keys and glasses can be put into a wallet, purse, or something else a person always wears or carries.

Q75. My husband paces around the house a lot. Is this bad for him or is it good exercise?

A75. Words like "wandering" and "pacing" are not easily defined. Many people with dementia do appear to walk about their home or a facility without a clear goal, but it is important to ask whether or why this is a problem.

Books and songs written about "wanderers" and "ramblin' men" often paint these actions in a positive light. I take this to mean that some people choose to walk about more than others, and that this is not necessarily negative. I dislike the term "wandering," because it has a negative connotation.

People with dementia who walk about when others do not might be bored, feel lost, or feel uncomfortable in an unfamiliar place. They might be looking for something or someone familiar, or be exercising.

You are more likely to find activities that the person can sit through and enjoy if you know what they enjoyed earlier in life and what they are able to enjoy now. It may take trial and error to find activities that engage them (*see Q46*). It may mean allowing a person to participate in an activity for just a few minutes, then get up and move around, and then encouraging them to return to the activity several minutes later.

It is quite possible that your husband is enjoying walking and exploring the environment. For people in a facility where there is no danger or negative impact on the quality of life of other residents, allowing the walking or moving about (not interfering with it) is often best. Family members are sometimes upset when they observe the person continually moving about. Educating them about the issue might help them understand that wandering is not necessarily a problem.

However, there are times when moving about places people at risk of harm or danger, or puts others at risk of harm. Examples include walking outside during bad weather, leaving home or a facility and being unable to find their way back, and walking in a place where there is a risk of being hit by a car, being assaulted, or being taken advantage of.

A very small number of people appear to be "driven pacers." These individuals walk constantly during their awake hours, do not stop even to eat, and appear restless. Attempts to engage them in activities are unsuccessful. They often are not able to sit with loved ones or other visitors. I think it likely that this rare occurrence is a brain-based symptom. I know of no intervention that changes driven pacing, so it should be tolerated unless it puts others at risk (for example, if the person bumps into frail people). Even if the person is at risk of harm from falling, the risk of harm from restraining them is often greater.

Antipsychotic medications can cause pacing and should be eliminated, if at all possible.

_____

Q76. My father has Alzheimer disease and doesn't recognize me. When I tell him that I am his oldest daughter, Jill, he becomes very upset and calls me a liar. He has lived with us for 2 years and this just started recently. How can this be, when he can still tell me what city he grew up in and what college he went to?

_____

A76. "Agnosia" is the word used to describe the inability to recognize the familiar even though vision is intact. Agnosia is one of the symptoms that usually develops in the second stage of Alzheimer disease (*see Q8*) and in people who have had a stroke in the right parietal lobe (*see the figure in Q18*). That your father knows where he grew up suggests that this is not a memory problem. He likely is able to tell you the names of all his children, further making the point that he has not forgotten he has children or who they are.

Some people are unable to recognize familiar objects such as a fork or their home, even though they have lived there for many years. Some people can see only one object at a time when there are several in their field of vision. For example, some people can see only one of several foods on their plate. Agnosia can be distinguished from forgetting because the person with agnosia can tell you about the person whose face they cannot recognize, describe details about the appearance of their home, or tell you what different foods look like.

Trying to convince your father of "the truth" will only make him more upset, because this information cannot correct his impaired ability to recognize you. Many people with this symptom are comfortable around loved ones even though they cannot specifically recognize them. Your father might recognize you by your voice but not your face.

Agnosia can be an especially upsetting symptom for caregivers. It may help to discuss your hurt with others who are understanding. Keeping in mind that this symptom does not reflect on his love for you won't make the upset go away but it might buffer it a little.

Q77. How do you differentiate incontinence from lack of recognition of where to go to the bathroom?

A77. By incontinence, I think you mean the inability to voluntarily control urination and bowel function. A person who develops incontinence should be assessed by a doctor or nurse to make sure it is not being caused by an infection or some other treatable problem. If that evaluation does not find a treatable cause, then you should focus on whether the problems associated with incontinence can be avoided.

Your question highlights the fact that there are multiple reasons adults might not be able to use the toilet correctly. People may have incontinence because they cannot find the toilet, cannot visually recognize a toilet, or are unable to sit on the toilet because they cannot visualize where the toilet is when their back is facing the toilet (as it is when we sit on a toilet seat), or because the parts of the brain that control voluntary urination and bowel evacuation have been destroyed by a brain disease.

The perception problems that develop in the middle stage of Alzheimer disease explain people's inability to accurately perceive the toilet (they do not know what they are seeing and so do not recognize it as a toilet) and people's inability to sit on the toilet when their back is towards it. They cannot form a mental picture of a toilet when they are not looking at it, and they are not able to lower their body to sit onto something they cannot see. These are examples of an *agnosia*, the inability to recognize a familiar object or to locate in space an object that one is not directly looking at (*see Q8 and Q76*).

People may be incontinent because they do not know where the bathroom is located, whether at home or in a facility. Interestingly, many people with Alzheimer disease can learn the location of the bathroom several weeks after moving to a new home or facility.

People, especially men, may urinate in pots or plants. This would suggest that they still have voluntary control but do not know where the bathroom is, cannot recognize a toilet, or do not know how to use a toilet.

Most people with advanced dementia lose the ability to voluntarily start and stop urination and bowel movements.

No matter what the cause, many people who have developed problems with urination and bowel movements can stay dry if they are put on a bathroom schedule. This means encouraging them or taking them to a bathroom every 2 hours. To determine if scheduling is going to help, it is imperative that the schedule be followed as strictly as possible. Every 2 or every 3 hours means exactly that. Realistically, you may not be able to do this at times, but it should be possible most of the time.

Some people with dementia and incontinence may not like being on a schedule or feel embarrassed and say they are being treated like a child. You are more likely to be successful if you are casual when you make the suggestion to go to the bathroom. The more you can make this natural—for example, "Since we're going to the supermarket, why don't you try going to the bathroom before we leave. You know how hard it is to walk all the way to the store bathroom."—the less likely it is to be taken as an insult.

> Encouraging people who are incontinent to use the toilet every 2 hours can help keep them dry during the day.

***

Q78. How can I get my husband to sleep better? How do I calm his fears in the middle of the night? His doctor has prescribed sleep medications, but they don't work.

***

A78. Disturbed sleep is common in dementia. As with any problematic issue, it is important to ask several questions.

1. Why is this a problem? Is it a problem for the person with dementia? A problem for the caregiver? A problem for others?

2. If the problem is causing distress for the person with dementia or placing that person at risk of harm, then it should be addressed. If it is a problem for the caregiver

but not for the person with dementia, it is reasonable to ask whether the caregiver is able to adapt to his sleep schedule. If the problem is affecting your ability to continue to care for your husband, then it should be identified as a problem and attempts should be made to address it.

3. What are the likely or potential causes of his disturbed sleep? Discussing this issue with a professional who is knowledgeable about dementia might help clarify whether it is related to some of the following:

   - *Medications or stimulating substances.* "Fluid pills" (diuretics) given in the evening or at bedtime can interrupt sleep by causing the person to awaken at night to urinate. Caffeine-containing drinks or foods eaten with or after dinner might be contributing to difficulty falling asleep. Some drugs given to enhance sleep may sedate a person but also suppress dreaming (REM) sleep and cause awakening in the middle of the night. Alcohol can do this, too, and also act as a diuretic. Antidepressant medications and anti-Alzheimer medications can cause vivid dreams that awaken people. If prescribed medications are possible causes, ask the person who prescribed them if they can be stopped, if the dose can be lowered, or if they can be given at a different time of the day. If they are not prescribed medications, make these changes on your own. If your husband is able to understand, talk with him about why you are making the decisions.

   - *Medical conditions* such as chronic heart failure can cause shortness of breath when lying down and interfere with sleep. Obstructive sleep apnea (OSA) causes frequent awakenings during the night when a person is asleep and leads to daytime drowsiness. Snoring is one symptom of OSA. Another is stopping breathing when asleep, often after a period of snoring.

- *Pain* due to a medical condition such as arthritis may be interfering with the ability to fall asleep or stay asleep, or may awaken the person early in the morning.

- *Lack of daytime activity.* Engaging in physical activity during the day can help people sleep better at night. However, not all people want to engage in activities. It is important to determine what the person enjoyed earlier in life and what they are able to participate in at the present time. Many people will participate in activities that meet these criteria, but not always. Respect the person's wishes but recognize that refusal is sometimes an indication that the person is being overwhelmed.

- *Anxiety* can cause difficulty falling asleep. In *depression*, people often are able to fall asleep normally but awaken in the middle of the night or early in the morning and be unable to get back to sleep (*see Q49*).

- A disorder called "*REM Sleep Behavior Disorder*" is associated with Lewy body dementia (*see Q16*). It is characterized by vivid dreams in which a person may become physically agitated, may kick or swing at a dreamed "attacker," and appear to others to be awake and frightened.

- *Alzheimer disease* can cause the death of brain cells in the area of the brain (called the "suprachiasmatic nucleus") that controls sleep. In my experience, patients whose sleep problems are related to damage in this area have a dramatically disturbed sleep/wake cycle—they sleep for several hours, then awaken for several hours, then sleep again, and then awaken. This often goes on for much of the day.

- Awakening and feeling that they are in an unfamiliar place.

General steps to try in addition to those mentioned above:

1. A person who awakens in a frightened state might have had a bad dream or awakened with the feeling that they are in an unfamiliar place. Reassuring them in a calm but confident manner ("You must have had a bad dream. We're at our house in Cincinnati and everything is OK.") might be enough to help them feel better and get back to sleep. Some people are more reassured by being hugged, stroked, or held.

2. If there is a potential medical disorder, talk with the person's doctor.

3. If a medication might be contributing to the sleep problem, discuss this with the person who has prescribed the drug and ask if other options are possible.

4. The person with REM sleep behavior disorder is safest if sleeping in a big bed without another person in the bed with them.

5. Some studies have shown that exposure to bright light during the morning or daytime improves nighttime sleep. While I am not convinced that daytime bright light exposure is effective in improving sleep, it should not be harmful unless it distresses the person who has dementia.

6. When the person is in a facility, allowing them to be awake at night and sleep when they do is usually the best approach if a daytime activity program doesn't help. If the person is at home and the caregiver's ability to function during the day is impaired or the caregiver's well-being is adversely affected, then a cautious trial of medication might be warranted.

7. No medications are FDA approved to treat sleep disorder in people with dementia, and there are no convincing studies demonstrating the efficacy of any medication for improving sleep in people with dementia. However, if all the above have been considered, *and* interventions based on them have not helped, *and* the problem persists, *and* if the person with dementia's inability to sleep at night is interfering with the family caregiver's well-being, a medication might be considered. In general, benzodiazepine sleep medications such as Ativan (lorazepam), Valium (diazepam) and Klonopin (clonazepam) are as likely to cause paradoxical worsening of sleep, memory, and behavior and to increase the risk of falls as they are to help, so I think they should be avoided if possible. Antipsychotic drugs increase the risk of death in people with dementia and it is my opinion that they should not be used as a sleep aid

unless there is some other symptom that requires their use (*see Q92*). Some doctors prescribe imidazopyridines (such as Ambien [zolpidem], Sonata [zaleplon], or Lunesta [eszopiclone]); melatonin; or the antidepressant trazodone, even though these drugs have not been shown to be effective. If a brief trial at an appropriate dose is unsuccessful, the drug should be discontinued. Again, studies have not shown these drugs to be beneficial in people with dementia.

Q79. What can I do when my husband, who is diagnosed with Alzheimer disease, demands to drink alcohol? If there is no alcohol in the house, he threatens to go buy it himself. Is he drinking because he wants to escape the thought that he has dementia, or because he can't remember how much he has consumed? The doctor said he could have 2 drinks a day to relax. Is he doing himself any harm physically? Will it make his dementia worse?

A79. The injured brain is more vulnerable to almost all drugs and medications. This is especially true of mind-altering substances that are taken to affect how people feel. It sounds as if your husband has been drinking alcohol for a long time. A few people begin drinking heavily as a result of dementia, and that raises different issues.

Since you discussed this with your doctor, I assume your husband is not having health problems as a result of his current alcohol intake. If he is, then his cutting back on the amount of alcohol he is drinking would be a higher priority.

Are there problems arising from his drinking now? Is he

more belligerent, aggressive, or tearful? Has it increased his risk of falls? Again, if any of these is true, then helping him cut back is a high priority.

If there are no obvious problems now and drinking is one of your husband's pleasures, then I would agree with your doctor. However, as the dementia progresses it is very likely that he will not be able to tolerate alcohol as he has in the past. You will need to control both how it gets into the house and how it is dispensed once in the house.

You may be able to call the store where he buys alcohol and get them to agree to stop selling to him. If you are able to control the amount he drinks you could try to serve fewer drinks or to water down the drinks you serve him.

Actions such as serving watered-down drinks are underhanded and deceptive, but they would allow him to have the pleasure of drinking while also lowering the risk. If he detects the dilution (this has happened with people I have cared for) and becomes upset, then you should not do it.

Treating alcoholism is difficult whether the person has dementia or not. You may have to consult an expert, but since he has dementia it is unlikely that any treatment program would be available to help him and you.

As with all decisions involving the care of people with dementia, you are doing what you can to maximize his quality of life and moderate his risk of harm. Over time the risk of harm may increase. If it does, you will need to be more restrictive, if you can. Right now, alcohol is a positive for his quality of life from his perspective. This supports allowing him to drink unless alcohol presents a danger.

Q80. My husband has fairly advanced Alzheimer disease and is not able to talk in full sentences. He looks sad and I worry he is depressed. How do you diagnose depression in a person who isn't able to understand questions about it?

A80. One of the challenges in identifying depression in people with dementia is that many people with dementia either cannot understand the questions they are being asked or cannot remember how they have been feeling in recent days or weeks. Family members, on the other hand, can often describe symptoms compatible with depression in their loved one.

Depression should be considered if a person:

- is eating less and losing weight and no other cause can be found (other causes of weight loss that should be considered include difficulty chewing food, difficulty swallowing food and liquids, and difficulty using eating utensils; dislike of the food they are being served; having many distractions at the eating table; cancer and heart failure);

- has become withdrawn and is not participating in activities that he previously enjoyed;

- has become less socially active;

- is crying frequently; or

- is making self-deprecating ("I'm a bad person") or self-blaming ("It's all my fault") comments.

_____

**Q81. My wife has Alzheimer disease and seems
depressed to me. She had an episode of depression
after the birth of our second child and seems the
same way now. Might counseling or medication help,
even though she has dementia?**

_____

A81. In my experience, people with early dementia who are
aware of their diagnosis can discuss their concerns and symptoms and may benefit from talking about them. Some people
with both dementia and clinical depression (*see Q80*) benefit
from increased stimulation, group participation, and physical
activity.

The studies of antidepressant medications as a treatment
for people with both dementia and depression have shown
mixed results. About half show a benefit and about half do not
(*see Q49*). If the symptoms of depression are severe, medication
should be considered, in my opinion, but the nonmedication
approaches should always be tried as well.

People who have had an episode of clinical depression prior
to developing dementia are at increased likelihood of becoming
depressed after their dementia develops.

_____

**Q82. My mother asks the same question over and over,
even within a minute. Is there anything I can do?**

_____

A82. Repeatedly saying the same thing, whether it is a question
or a statement, usually reflects severe memory impairment.
The person does not remember having just asked the question
or making the statement. It can also reflect language impair-

ment if the person with dementia is unable to talk in complete sentences or have a conversation in which there is the usual "back and forth."

Repetition may also reflect boredom or fear of being alone, or it may be a way for people with dementia to combat the worry and anxiety that accompany not knowing where they are or what is happening next.

There are several things to try. For people who are worried or anxious, try reassuring them that everything is fine and that you are taking care of things. You might ask them if they are afraid or worried, but if that upsets them further, try other strategies.

Boredom can be counteracted by trying to engage the person in activities such as going on a walk, talking with others in a group, playing a game, or having a conversation about issues they enjoy, such as what the grandchildren are doing. Previously enjoyed activities are more likely to engage people than activities they have never done before.

Gently moving the focus of the conversation to a topic related to whatever they are repeating might help. For example, if the person keeps asking when her mother is coming to pick her up, ask her about her favorite memory of her mother or talk about some other issue that involves her mother, such as your favorite remembrance (even if her mother is deceased).

Breaking a cycle of repetition sometimes requires lying. The ethics of this is discussed in *Q88, Q96, Q97*, and *Q98*.

Q83. I work in a nursing home. How can we tell when people with severe dementia are in pain? Does dementia cause hypersensitivity or lack of sensitivity to pain?

A83. Pain is an important issue, whether the person is at home or in long-term care. The common causes of dementia do not impair or lessen the ability to experience pain, but *detecting* it can be challenging. What dementia does impair is people's ability to express that they are in pain, to describe what they are feeling, and to recognize what is bothering them. If they have had a stroke that affects sensation, they may have a diminished or increased ability to experience pain in one part of the body.

People with dementia may not be able to say that they are in pain, describe what time of day it occurs, or describe where their pain is located. Therefore, caregivers must be attuned to the possibility that people with dementia who are crying, not moving a body part, becoming less involved in activities, becoming more irritable, or striking out, may be in pain. This means it is important to ask every person with dementia who is exhibiting any of these signs whether they are in pain. They may be able to respond accurately but might not. If a person appears to be "guarding" or not moving a body part, ask their permission to touch and gently move it. If the person grimaces, then further investigation is indicated. Look for bruises or other evidence of an injury.

If the person is in a facility, inform the staff and ask that a medical professional examine the person. If the person is at home and pain is a possibility, notify a medical practitioner. A thorough physical examination can detect and localize pain.

I have had patients who may have been in pain, but neither the family, other staff, nor I could be sure. Attempts to soothe them, redirect them, engage them, or otherwise involve them failed. Such situations are uncommon, but when they happen, a trial of an analgesic (pain medication) is worthwhile. Giving the person several doses of acetaminophen (Tylenol) or ibuprofen (such as Motrin), if not contraindicated, is one way to assess if a noncommunicative or agitated person is in pain. A cautious trial of a low-dose opiate is occasionally appropriate.

Q84. My husband sometimes cries suddenly, especially when we are in public. Why does this happen and can I do anything to help him feel better?

A84. Sudden crying can indicate pain, depression, fear, or a sense of being overwhelmed (see Q78, Q80, Q81, Q82, and Q83). Ask yourself if the crying always occurs in a specific circumstance. This might identify the trigger.

If pain or depression is a possibility, talk with his doctor. If he appears frightened or overwhelmed before he cries, think about changing the environment so it is less stressful, more supportive, and more attuned to his needs.

In addition, a disorder called "pseudobulbar affect (PBA)," sometimes referred to as "emotional incontinence," can occur in people with brain damage due to dementia, brain trauma, multiple sclerosis, multiple strokes, or ALS (amyotrophic lateral sclerosis). PBA is characterized by sudden crying or laughing. Sometimes there is a trigger but sometimes not. If there is a trigger, the crying or laughter is often out of proportion to whatever is stimulating it. Many people who have PBA describe their crying or laughing as "more extreme" than they are actually feeling and will say that it is not a genuine reflection of what they are experiencing. Many of these individuals can identify a trigger, for example, the national anthem, a sad scene in a movie, or a photograph of a familiar person, but still say that they are not feeling as upset as they look. Some people have easily teared up all their lives, and for them this is normal.

Explaining that this is a symptom of their illness helps some people accept it and be less distressed by it. Others complain of being embarrassed by the expression of this extreme emotion. One medication, Neudexta (dextromethorphan/quinidine), has been approved by the FDA to treat this condition. While not FDA approved to treat PBA, standard antidepressants can also diminish or abolish frequent crying in some people and may be less expensive.

Q85. My mother has pretty advanced Alzheimer disease. I try to visit her at least twice a week but am at a loss about what to say to her. Having a real conversation is hard. Any suggestions?

A85. When I was first learning about Alzheimer disease, I came across an article by geriatric psychiatrist Jack Weinberg titled "What Do I Say to My Mother When I Have Nothing to Say?" In the article Dr. Weinberg answered his own question. He wrote that he came to realize that the most important things to his mother were his visits and the fact that he and she were talking to each other, not the specific content of their conversations. He also realized that repeatedly having the same conversation might be boring to him, but it was not to his mother. She loved hearing about the grandchildren, about his current work, and about other events in his life, even if they had talked about it 5 minutes or 5 days ago.

Dr. Weinberg's observations helped me realize the value of seeing things from the perspective of the person with dementia. Having a conversation is what is pleasurable at that moment. Whether the person remembers that they had a similar conversation recently is unimportant. People with severe memory impairment are "living in the moment." For them, interacting with people is their greatest source of pleasure. This can help overcome feelings of being alone, lost, or in an unfamiliar place. Your mother may not remember that you had visited earlier in the day or yesterday, but she will know, while you are talking with her, that you are her daughter and that you are important to, and enjoy, each other.

> **Often, what is most important to a person with dementia is visits from loved ones, not the specific content of their conversations.**

Q86. What can I do to deflect or redirect my wife's infidelity accusations?

A86. Unfortunately, this is a relatively common symptom. In fact, Dr. Alzheimer's initial patient had this symptom. She became increasingly distressed and physically aggressive, and these were the triggers that led her husband to bring her to a doctor for an evaluation.

I assume the accusations are false. Unfortunately, it is sometimes impossible to convince others that this is the case. However, there are often aspects of the ill person's complaint which show that the accusation is a symptom of an illness and not true. For example, one patient I treated with this symptom repeatedly told me that she knew her husband was having an ongoing affair because she saw wrinkles in the blanket on their bed almost every day.

I also assume that, like the husband of Dr. Alzheimer's first patient, you have told your wife that her concerns are not true. If you have not done so, it is reasonable to do so once or twice, just to convince yourself that this doesn't help. It is also worth trying to change the subject, have her engage in activities with others, enroll her in day care, and even tell her that the infidelity has stopped.

In Q88, Q96, Q97, and Q98, I discuss some of the ethical challenges that arise when we lie to a person or don't directly address their concerns, correct incorrect ideas, or address repeated complaints.

Part of the challenge of the symptom you are describing is that the person with dementia who is making the accusation is often repeatedly telling others about it—children, friends, neighbors, and professional caregivers. I think it is OK to tell these individuals, in private, that your wife's accusations are not true but are a symptom of her illness. Tell them that you are trying to shield her from the distress that these thoughts are causing and could use their help. I suggest telling them it is OK for them to tell her that they will ask you about it, to tell her that they will look into it, or to comment on how distressed she looks. If any of these replies stop her from making the accusations (usually temporarily) or seem to help her calm down, then that is the best that can be done.

Rarely, these beliefs lead to physical aggression. If this happens repeatedly and her concerns cannot be deflected, then

> Untrue accusations of infidelity are common. If telling the person once or twice that it is untrue doesn't help, try to
> * change the subject;
> * distract the person by engaging them in another activity;
> * enroll them in day care; or
> * tell them that the infidelity has stopped.
>
> If you find something that works, do that whenever you need to, if you can.

a very cautious trial of medication might be necessary. If the symptom occurs only when you are present, and her distress cannot be relieved, then you might need to spend less time with her.

It is also important for you to get your own support. Accusations like this hurt. Being able to talk to someone (a friend, family member, clergy, or mental health professional) about your hurt, frustration, sadness, and loss (of her companionship, for example) doesn't make the problem go away, but it can help you from becoming overwhelmed by it.

Q87. My husband was always gentle and calm. Now he gets angry at the drop of a hat. Are there things I can do to address his anger issues?

A87. About 30% of people with Alzheimer disease undergo what people describe as a change in personality. I'm not always sure what this phrase means, since some people seem to be themselves in many situations but different in the way you have described.

If your husband is himself in many situations but becomes easily angered, you are describing what is sometimes referred to as a "catastrophic reaction." This term refers to the fact that the person seems to be reacting as if there were a major catastrophe when the trigger was either minor or indiscernible. Catastrophic reactions are common in people with all types of brain disease. They reflect a problem with modulating or tamping down emotional responses. They are thought to reflect damage to the frontal lobes (*see the figure in Q18*), the part of the brain that assesses social circumstances, helps us use thinking processes to control our emotions, and contributes to mental flexibility in the face of challenges.

Catastrophic reactions usually develop quickly. They are characterized by facial flushing, verbal expressions of anger (including yelling), and, sometimes, physical expressions of anger such as pushing or striking out.

The triggers of catastrophic reactions differ from person to person. They can seem quite minor but are overwhelming for that person. If triggers can be anticipated, do your best to avoid them, but recognize that this is not always possible. Examples of triggers that are sometimes unavoidable are necessary daily routines, medical care, and avoidance of unsafe situations. In addition, environmental stimuli such as a siren or a crying baby can trigger a catastrophic reaction.

Catastrophic reactions can sometimes be detected at the very beginning, especially by a caregiver who knows the person well. Early manifestations of a catastrophic reaction include facial flushing, restlessness, mumbling, or signs of distress.

If the triggers cannot be anticipated, avoided, or minimized, or if a catastrophic reaction has already begun, its severity can be lessened or minimized by distracting the person or removing them from the situation. The care provider should remain calm but in charge. It usually helps to reassure the person that you recognize the problem, that you are addressing it, and that they will be safe. Care providers should avoid raising their voice, grabbing the person, appearing frightened, or acting overwhelmed. Some people with catastrophic reactions are helped if their emotional upset is acknowledged, but others are made worse by commenting on their distress.

It is not always possible to avoid the events that trigger a catastrophic reaction. Steps that may help abort the reaction or minimize its severity include
- removing the triggering stressor,
- redirecting the person's attention to something else,
- remaining calm and not becoming distressed, and
- reassuring the person that the problem is being taken care of.

Q88. My wife cries almost every afternoon because she thinks her mother should be picking her up and is late. When I tell her that her mother died 25 years ago, she becomes even more upset and often begins to cry.

A88. The term "sundowning" is often used to describe the regular occurrence of distress and agitation in the late afternoon or evening. Interestingly, it has been very hard for researchers to verify that distress and agitation occur more often at one time of day than another.

It is less important to prove that sundowning exists than it is to help people who are reported to have this problem. Potential causes include boredom, fatigue in the person with dementia, fatigue in the caregiver, lower staffing ratios in the afternoon and evening, and more noise and stimulation later in the day because visitors tend to come later in the day. I doubt that lower light levels play a major role, because there is no evidence that sundowning occurs later in the day during the summer, when it stays light outside much later.

You might try to:

- schedule her for more activities around the time she usually becomes upset,

- have her take a nap around the time she seems to become upset,

- expose her to more light (a few studies have found that more light decreases behavioral problems), and

- minimize the number of visitors, medical visits, trips, and other forms of stimulation at that time.

I recommend trying one approach at a time, because that makes it easier to determine what doesn't work and what does.

It almost never helps to "correct" the person (for example, "Dear, don't you remember? Your mother has been dead for 25 years."). See *Q96*, *Q97*, and *Q98* for more discussion of this issue.

Q89. My husband has been in an assisted living facility for 6 months. For the past month he has been spending all his time with one female resident. They often walk the halls holding hands and talking to each other. Lately, he doesn't even seem to know me when I visit. I am sure that he was faithful to me during our 45-year marriage, so this is a shock. What should I do?

A89. I can understand your surprise and hurt. It is likely that he does not recognize you because he has the symptom called "agnosia," in which people are *not able* to recognize familiar faces, places, or objects (*see Q8 and Q76*). If this is the case, telling him who you are will not help. His "ignoring" you is not a purposeful action. It is a reflection of his inability to recognize who you are.

He may still enjoy your visits, even if he does not know exactly who you are. If he does not interact with you or always becomes upset, then you might have to decrease the frequency of your visits. If you have to do this, I encourage you to touch base with the staff regularly to make sure he is being well cared for.

In my experience the ability to recognize familiar people sometimes comes and goes, especially when it is a new symptom. He might recognize you one time and not another. When he does not recognize you, I recommend limiting the time you are there—this will be better for both of you.

In some ways you are experiencing a double loss. Your husband has been changed by his dementia and your marriage has been taken from you. Discussing your feelings with family, friends, staff, or a professional counselor may help.

Q90. My father is very ill with cancer and likely to die soon. My mother, who has had Alzheimer disease for 4 or 5 years, seems unaware of this, and we haven't brought it up. Should we discuss his illness with her now? If he dies, will she remember that? If she doesn't remember, should we keep reminding her?

A90. Grieving is a long-term process. Most people need to talk about potential or actual losses and feel comforted by the ability to do so with people they are close to. If your mother has not noticed that her husband is ill, it is likely but not definite that her unawareness is coming from her illness. Nonetheless, I think she should be told how ill he is, because we cannot be sure what she does and doesn't know. You can use her response to guide you in what to do next. If she becomes upset and is able to talk about her feelings, then she should be supported, listened to, and empathized with as you would anyone in that situation. If she isn't able to understand what you are telling her, denies that he is ill, or repeatedly becomes upset and is unable to talk about her feelings, you should stop bringing it up.

I would approach the question of what to say to her after your father's death in a similar fashion. Informing her when it happens, as you would anyone, seems appropriate. If she forgets quickly, repeatedly becomes distressed when you remind her of his death and then again forgets it several minutes later, or seems unable to talk about it, it is likely that her illness has robbed her of the ability to grieve.

Many people with dementia, even advanced dementia, seem to have some remembrance of a significant loss, even though they are vague on details. This awareness might come out during a conversation, even if they are unable to retrieve the information when asked directly. If this is the case, I recommend using their reaction as a guide for what to do next. If you say something like, "I really miss Dad a lot, too," and your mother becomes very agitated, I would be hesitant to continue the conversation. Helping her calm down by holding her hand, hugging her, just being with her, or changing the subject might be best. If she becomes tearful, seems to understand, and seems to be benefiting from the discussion, then proceed as you would with anyone in this difficult time. In the end, you should do what seems best for your mother's emotional well-being.

Q91. Why do people with dementia develop swallowing problems?

A91. Swallowing requires the coordination of muscles in the mouth and throat and requires the closing off of the breathing tube (trachea) and the opening of the swallowing tube (esophagus). The centers of the brain that control these functions are located in the brain stem, which is at the bottom of the brain (*see the figure in Q18*).

Most progressive dementias either directly damage the areas of the brain that initiate and coordinate swallowing or they damage fibers that come into those areas of the brain from above. This happens earlier in some diseases than others.

When the swallowing mechanism becomes paralyzed or uncoordinated, liquids and solids can go into the lungs (because the trachea has not been correctly closed off) instead of down the esophagus. This is referred to as "aspiration." Aspiration can lead to pneumonia due to chemical irritation or infection.

If a stroke damages the swallowing control system, swallowing problems develop immediately. Since most dementias progress slowly, the swallowing problems they cause develop gradually. At first a person might choke occasionally, especially on thin fluids like water or on poorly chewed food. Secretions are constantly being produced in the nose and mouth, and these might also stimulate coughing when they go into the breathing system. Some people have reflux, a regurgitation of stomach contents up the esophagus, which can lead to aspiration.

Speech and language pathologists can evaluate a person's aspiration risk and advise steps that can be taken to lessen this risk, including the use of thickened liquids and pureed food. These may lessen the risk of aspiration, but they cannot fully prevent it. Feeding tubes do not prevent aspiration, either.

Q92. Why do people with dementia lose the ability to walk?

A92. In Alzheimer disease, the brain cells directly controlling the muscles of the legs are not impaired, but the pathways that connect these cells to other parts of the brain become damaged. Walking ability gradually declines as these connecting pathways are destroyed.

Early impairment of balance can occur in Parkinson disease (Q17), whether or not dementia develops, and in dementia with Lewy bodies (Q16). Progressive supranuclear palsy (PSP) and cortico-basal degeneration (CBD) can also impair walking early in the disease. In vascular dementia, strokes either directly kill the cells that control leg movement or impair the pathways involved in walking. As a result, walking difficulty due to vascular brain disease usually develops suddenly.

Normal pressure hydrocephalus (NPH) causes unsteady walking, urinary incontinence, and dementia. These symptoms often begin within 6 months of the first symptom. Importantly, NPH can be treated if recognized early. Any person who develops unsteady walking within the first year of developing symptoms of dementia should be assessed for NPH.

Any person who develops unsteady walking within the first year of developing symptoms of dementia should be assessed for normal pressure hydrocephalus, which can be treated if recognized early.

7

What Are Some of the Difficult Decisions Caregivers Face?

Q93. I'm worried about my father's memory. He repeats himself 2 or 3 times in an hour, and if I tell him he's already told me the same thing, he just brushes it off. I told him I thought he should talk to his doctor about it, but he says there's nothing wrong. What should I do now?

A93. The first question to ask yourself is how dangerous the situation is at present. If he is driving and has had several accidents or if he keeps forgetting to take medication and has been hospitalized as a result, then you are morally justified to act in ways that might help him, even if he resists.

However, from your description there does not appear to be any clear danger now. If that is correct, I suggest you express your concern to him again in a few weeks and enlist the support of your sisters and brothers if you have any. Perhaps he will follow through if several people express concern.

It might be helpful to express your concern to him in a way that is not threatening or insulting. Perhaps he would be willing to raise the issue with his doctor if you say, "Would you do it for me, so I won't worry? I'll feel better even if you're right and I'm wrong."

If he still refuses and your concerns persists, I suggest that every few weeks you repeat your observations and again suggest that he be evaluated.

> When trying to encourage people who believe there is nothing wrong with their memory to be evaluated, it may help to express concern in a way that is not threatening or insulting. You might say, "Would you do it for me, so I won't worry? I'll feel better even if you're right and I'm wrong."

Q94. Once the diagnosis of dementia has been made, should the person be told, even if he or she denies having a problem?

A94. In the United States we believe that people's health information is theirs. This means that a doctor should inform all patients of their diagnosis.

About one-third of people with Alzheimer disease are not aware that they are having problems (*see Q62*). When told of the diagnosis, many of these individuals will deny having any problems with memory or thinking, or they may ascribe any difficulties they are having to normal aging with statements such as, "I'm just like all my friends."

One way to think about this is to recognize that people have a "right not to know" a diagnosis. Although rare, there are people who choose not to know. In Alzheimer disease, though, most people who downplay or outright deny having cognitive problems lack the ability to recognize their limitations. I am convinced that this is a symptom of the disease in the majority of these individuals, because unawareness or denial of memory impairment is much less common in people with similar levels of disability caused by dementias other than Alzheimer disease.

When I newly diagnose dementia, I first inform patients that I am concerned about their memory and would like to discuss it with them. If they disagree that a memory or thinking problem is present or if they deny having any difficulty, I say to them something like, "I would like to inform you of my opinion." If they still insist that there is no problem and act as if they do not want to have a discussion, then I stop. I will repeat this discussion at the next visit, but I believe it is improper to force a person to listen. For me, honoring the person's wishes is important, and I take their denial as a sign that they either do not want to know or lack the ability to recognize their impairment.

> In people with dementia, denial of illness is a sign that they are unable to recognize their impairments, either because the disease blocks their self-awareness or because they do not want to know.

However, if the disease blocks a person's ability to recognize that they are in danger, I have a duty to protect that person. Therefore, I do my best to ensure that someone in the family or a close friend is informed when this is possible. On the rare occasion that such a person is not available, or if the person refuses to allow me to discuss my findings with others, I make an assessment of the dangerousness of their current situation.

If I believe there is danger—for example, if the person seems unable to take prescribed and necessary medication, has become lost walking or driving, or seems at risk of being taken advantage of financially—I may have to inform the state agency whose job it is to protect such individuals. These agencies go by names such as "adult protective services." HIPAA (Health Insurance Portability and Accountability Act) regulations do not allow sharing of health information with others without a person's permission, but if danger appears likely, then a professional can notify the appropriate agency.

Most older people who come to a doctor do so with another person. I have never had the experience that the patient does not want me to talk with that person.

Q95. My father lives alone and was diagnosed with Alzheimer disease last week. As far as I can tell, he is doing OK. The house is neat and he hasn't lost weight. Should I talk with him about moving to a place where he can receive help once he needs it, or should I wait until he starts having problems?

A95. Since your father has shared his diagnosis with you, it seems natural to begin by asking him his thoughts about the diagnosis and about how he is doing. Openly talking about a diagnosis of dementia is similar to talking to people about other serious medical illnesses such as cancer. Although some individuals worry that they will "make things worse" for the person with the illness by bringing up bad news, experience teaches that most people welcome the discussion.

If your father is open to talking about his diagnosis, I would ask whether he has thoughts regarding his future needs and if he has already taken steps to address them. He may surprise you and tell you about plans or thoughts you were unaware of. If he says he has not made any plans, I suggest asking whether he has thought about "papers"—writing a will and filling out durable power of attorney documents. If he has not done both of these and is not planning on doing so, tell him you would like to help him think about his options or, if he prefers, help him find someone who can advise him.

If his plans are vague, you can be supportive of what he has done thus far and tell him you will help him think more about his preferences for the future. Since he may not be aware of the range of options, you might ask if he knows what the possibilities are.

If he does not want to discuss these issues, I suggest saying that you want to be supportive and that you will bring them up in the future. You might ask if there is someone else he would be more comfortable talking to about these issues. If you are the only person available with whom he can discuss his plans, I suggest trying to leave the issue open for future discussion by saying something like, "I hope we can talk about it later."

Giving up a home is psychologically difficult for many people. Most people have emotional connections to their home and neighborhood. In addition, moving may symbolize loss of independence, loss of the familiar, and a loss of linkages to one's past.

Moving also raises many practical difficulties such as identifying the available options, sifting through complicated financial issues, choosing among and discarding long-cherished possessions, finding a new doctor, and adapting to a scheduled day. The difficulties and stresses associated with moving are often magnified by the cognitive changes that accompany dementia. Changes in executive function (*see Q8 and Q18*) can make it harder to make choices, to think ahead, and to keep one's emotions appropriate to the situation. Some people will welcome help, but others strongly resist it. Openly acknowledging these emotional, financial, practical, and cognitive barriers can make it easier for some people to accept help.

Q96. My mother has had Alzheimer disease for 6 or 7 years and I have been a widow for almost 4 years. I see her almost every day. Last week for the first time she asked why my husband hadn't come to see her lately and then said, "I guess he's been busy at work." If this happens again should I tell her the truth, that he died 4 years ago, or just agree with her?

A96. You raise a difficult ethical question. Is it right to lie to a person with dementia?

Most people agree that lying is wrong and that truth telling is the way we want to act, especially with people we care about. The challenge raised by dementia is that what is true for the person with dementia is not necessarily true for anyone else. What should be done when people mistakenly believe that their parents are alive, that someone will be picking them up and taking them home, or that family members do not visit them?

Most of the time this issue comes up after someone has already told the person with dementia "the truth" and been met with disbelief or distress because the person with dementia did not know that a person they love had died, that they are now living in a facility rather than their home, or that a family member had visited several hours before. If the person with dementia has not been told the truth, I believe this should be done. Their response might surprise you.

The real challenge here is, whose "truth" are we to accept? Unfortunately, the person with dementia is not able to remember what is "true" for everyone else, so for them they have had no visitors, their parents are still alive, and someone has stolen money from them. If the person with dementia lacks the ability to know the truth, then correcting them or "telling them the truth," which is many people's instinct, cannot benefit them. This is very unfortunate, because it means that the person with dementia is unable to grieve the loss of loved ones or to accept the difficulty of a move away from their home.

> If the person with dementia lacks the ability to know the truth, then correcting them or "telling them the truth," which is many people's instinct, cannot benefit them.

Because the person with dementia lacks the ability to accept what others know to be true, I conclude it is best if others see the issue from the perspective of the person with dementia. This means accepting that they cannot know what we know and that they cannot benefit from what we know to be the truth. In fact, their truth *is* the truth for them.

Some people want to call this "fibbing," "telling a white lie," or "entering their world" rather than use the word "lying." I believe it is important to acknowledge *to ourselves* that we are lying when we tell mistruths such as "Your mother went to visit her parents and will be back Monday" or "I can understand how lonely you must be because no one has visited lately. I'll try to talk with your family about visiting more often." I believe that acknowledging to ourselves that we are lying makes it less likely that lying will bleed into other areas of our life. If we feel bad but know it is the right thing to do for the person with dementia, then we are more likely to hold true to our dislike for lying. This is the type of issue for which there is no single "right" answer. Talking with others who have had similar experiences, for example, professionals who have advised other people in this circumstance or members of a support group, and using the person with dementia as the determinant of what is right to do, might be helpful in deciding how to best handle these difficult situations.

Q97. You say it is OK to lie or mislead (see Q88 and Q96), but what can I say when my husband tells me I haven't visited him in weeks when, in fact, I have been there at least once a day for the past 6 months?

A97. It is certainly appropriate to tell him, "You might not remember, because you're having trouble with your memory, but I did come by yesterday." My guess is that this information will either upset him, make him feel reprimanded, or not convince him that you are visiting regularly. If that doesn't help him, I think it is more reassuring for you to say, "I'll try to do better" or "I plan on being here every afternoon for the next few weeks."

It sometimes helps to acknowledge the feelings behind such a statement, but there is a risk that doing so will upset him also. You could see what happens if you say, "I know you are feeling lonely. Do you want to talk about it?" and see how that goes.

Correcting him also serves no purpose, at least from his perspective. It emphasizes his impairment and doesn't offer

It sometimes helps to acknowledge the feelings behind the misstatements of a person who has dementia.

a solution. I think you want to directly or indirectly indicate your love and support, and let him know he is not being abandoned. Of course you are not abandoning him, but, because of his memory impairment, he cannot remember that you come regularly, that he enjoys your visits while you are there, or that he has a memory disorder.

Q98. My mother is in her late 70s and was diagnosed with Alzheimer disease 5 or 6 years ago. Many of her friends and relatives are dying and I am not sure whether I should tell her when someone she was close to dies. My sister and father say she has a right to know and that it is in her best interest to tell her. What do you think?

A98. Reasons to share bad news include allowing grieving to begin, offering support, and sharing memories and plans. How has your mother responded when told about the deaths of friends and family thus far? Does she become upset and unable to talk or does she reminisce and express her feelings? If she is not harmed by the discussion, then telling her is reasonable, as long as you realize that there is a good chance she will not remember that the person has died. If she is unable to remember the death, she will not be able to grieve the loss.

If she repeatedly talks about people who have died as if they are alive, then I see no benefit in reminding her that the person is dead. A better response might be to ask your mother about her memories of the person and to talk about your memories of the person. If appropriate, you can say that you miss the person. While I prefer to err on the side of sharing too much, it is only appropriate to do so if the person is not harmed, even in the short run.

Q99. Who can decide that a person is incompetent to make their own health decisions?

A99. As a general rule, "incompetency" is a legal term meaning that a judge has determined that a person temporarily or permanently lacks the ability to make decisions. In the United States, adults, defined as either age 18 or 21, automatically gain competency. Although only a judge can take away an adult's freedom to make choices for themselves, all jurisdictions have rules that also allow physicians, psychologists, and some other mental health practitioners to determine that a person lacks the capacity to make important decisions.

One reason durable powers of attorney for finances and health (see Q59) are so important is that they provide the means for a person to determine, while they have the capacity to do so, who should represent their wishes if they become incompetent. Many jurisdictions provide other ways, such as legally binding checklists, by which people can indicate what medical treatments they would want if they became incompetent.

Q100. How do you decide when to treat a newly diagnosed terminal illness in a person with dementia?

A100. If the person with dementia is competent to make decisions about his medical care, then the fact that he has dementia is not relevant. All adults in this circumstance should make their own decisions.

If the person is not competent and they have a durable power of attorney for health, then their substitute decision maker should determine from their advance directive or living will whether they have made their wishes explicit. If they did, then their prior wish should generally be followed. If there is no explicit discussion of treating a terminal illness and the substitute decision maker does not have direct knowledge of what the person would have wanted, then the substitute decision maker should try to determine, based on the person's values before they became ill, what the person would have wanted had they been able to make the decision.

Q101. My mother has had Alzheimer disease for almost 9 years, is no longer able to speak or feed herself, has lost 12 pounds in 4 months, and pushes people away when they try to feed her. Her doctor has asked us whether we want to place a feeding tube. I am her durable power of attorney for health. What advice do you have for me?

A101. This is a morally challenging issue because it is more than a medical decision. For many people, feeding those who are unable to feed themselves is a basic human value. On the other hand, it is not clear that feeding tubes provide any medical benefit for people with advanced dementia.

From your description, your mother is unable to give consent, so the decision falls to you as her durable power of attorney. If your mother indicated what her wishes would be in a power of attorney document or living will, or had a discussion, while competent, with you, then her wishes should be followed.

If she never indicated what she would want, you should consider the following medical facts. First, in people with advanced dementia feeding tubes do not prolong life or prevent pneumonia (*see Q37*). Second, percutaneous endoscopic gastrostomy (PEG) feeding tubes, which are placed through the abdominal wall directly into the stomach, are uncomfortable for some people, causing them to constantly tug on the tube. Third, feeding tubes deprive people of the pleasure of taste and eating unless they are also able to take in some food or liquid by mouth.

Even if she has not expressed a specific wish about this circumstance, you might be able to infer what she would have decided based on her lifelong values and on the medical facts. For many people who are asked to make this decision for another, the most challenging issue is whether the person for whom the decision is being made will suffer. There is no scientific answer to this question, but I have been through the experience with a number of patients with end-stage dementia and offer the following observations. People losing weight from dementia do so over months, that is, gradually. If their fluid intake is not adequate, they gradually become dehydrated but do not appear thirsty or uncomfortable. Also, I have talked with cognitively normal people who recovered from being dehydrated, and they have not recalled feeling thirsty. These observations lead me to conclude that people who gradually lose weight and become dehydrated do not suffer discomfort.

You should not be rushed into a hasty decision. Discuss the issues with others in the family, talk openly about any difficulties you are having in making the decision, and be open about your feelings. Feel free to talk with people who might help, such as her doctor, clergy, and friends who have been in the same situation.

Index

Page numbers in *italics* indicate illustrations.

family members, recognition of,
99–100
feeding skills, 14
feeding tubes, 70, 124, 137–39
finances, durable power of attorney
for, 78
free recall memory, 1
frontal lobes, 118
frontotemporal dementia (FTD),
10, 25–27, 52
frustration: of caregivers, 87; from
language impairments, 93–94
future plans, discussing, 83–84,
130–31

galantamine (Razadyne), 61–64
gender, as risk factor, 48
gene testing kits, 36
genetics as cause of Alzheimer
disease, 34–38, 49
ginkgo, 65
glucose PET scans, 16
granulovacuolar degeneration, 26
grief, 122–23, 133
guilt of caregivers, 57, 87

Haldol (haloperidol), 66
harm reduction, 108
head trauma and CTE, 28–29
health, durable power of attorney
for, 78, 137–39
Health App, 97
Health Insurance Portability and
Accountability Act (HIPAA), 130
help at home, finding, 89–90
hematomas, subdural, 16, 22
hemorrhagic strokes, 27
hereditary, Alzheimer disease as,
34–38, 49
herpes virus infections, 42
high blood pressure, 45

HIPAA (Health Insurance Portability and Accountability Act),
130
hippocampus, 50
home: finding help for, 89–90;
giving up, 131
hospice care, 70–71
hospitals and delirium, 90–91

imidazopyridines, 107
incidence rate, 49
incompetence: determination of,
136; power of attorney documents and, 77–78; refusal to
take medications and, 95–96;
treatment of terminal illnesses
and, 137
incontinence, 100–102
independence, tips for maximizing,
14
infection, links between Alzheimer
disease and, 41–42
infidelity, accusations of, 115–17
information: learning new, 51,
96–97; retrieval of, 1

jellyfish protein, 65–66

language impairments, 9, 12–14,
93–94
language variant of FTD, 26
lawyers, consulting with, 77
learning new information, 51,
96–97
Lewy bodies, 10
Lewy body dementia, 23, 104, 124
light exposure, 106, 120
living in moment, 115
living wills, 78
lobes of brain, 25
locator chips, 97